Values-Based Health
and Social Care

Values-Based Health and Social Care

Beyond Evidence-Based Practice

Edited by
Jill McCarthy and Pat Rose

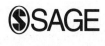

Los Angeles | London | New Delhi
Singapore | Washington DC

First published 2010

SAGE Publications Ltd
1 Oliver's Yard
55 City Road
London EC1Y 1SP

SAGE Publications Inc.
2455 Teller Road
Thousand Oaks, California 91320

SAGE Publications India Pvt Ltd
B 1/I 1 Mohan Cooperative Industrial Area
Mathura Road
New Delhi 110 044

SAGE Publications Asia-Pacific Pte Ltd
33 Pekin Street #02-01
Far East Square
Singapore 048763

Library of Congress Control Number: 2009943064

British Library Cataloguing in Publication data

A catalogue record for this book is available from the British Library

ISBN 978-1-84860-201-4
ISBN 978-1-84860-202-1 (pbk)

Typeset by C&M Digitals (P) Ltd, Chennai, India
Printed and bound in Great Britain by TJ International Ltd, Padstow, Cornwall
Printed on paper from sustainable resources

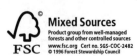

Mixed Sources
Product group from well-managed
forests and other controlled sources
www.fsc.org Cert no. SGS-COC-2482
© 1996 Forest Stewardship Council
FSC

Contents

About the Authors

Dr Jillian McCarthy is an experienced educationalist having worked in the higher education sector for the last 18 years. She is a qualified nurse and maintains an interest in matters relating to nursing, health and wellbeing. She has a particular interest in the education of health professionals particularly in regard to learning technologies and has published and presented in this field. Her interest in values-based health care has developed over the last few years having noticed unease amongst health and social care professionals in regard to a sole reliance on evidence-based practice. It is her intention that this book will go someway towards addressing this issue.

Pat Rose was a Senior Lecturer at the University of Chester until her retirement in 2009. She contributed to undergraduate and post-graduate programmes within the Faculty of Health and Social Care and had a particular interest in practice learning and innovation in care provision both in hospital and community settings. Her professional background was in general children's nursing and health visiting.

Pat has published widely in subjects including, ethics, child health, research methods, and pedagogy. In her retirement she is supporting inexperienced writers as they embark on an academic career. She is also is active in the organisation 'City of Sanctuary' which is a movement seeking to build a culture of hospitality for people seeking sanctuary in the UK.

Pauline Alexander is a Senior Lecturer within the Faculty of Health and Social Care at the University of Chester. She has worked in Higher Education since 1982. She joined the University of Chester from the University of Liverpool where she had been Director of Studies in Continuing Professional Development, Director of Studies Bachelor of Nursing (Hons), and Examinations and Assessments Officer. Pauline has worked within the NHS in Accident and Emergency Care, High Dependency, General Surgery, Care of the Elderly and Primary Care. She was the Lead Researcher on an NHS North West Region Research and Development grant, undertaking a study into patient's perceptions of telephone triage. She is currently the Programme

Leader for the BSc Community Health Studies and is involved in teaching Non-Medical Prescribing, Work-based Learning Modules and Pre–Registration Nursing.

Julie Bailey- McHale   worked initially in mental health nursing in the acute inpatient sector. Since moving to higher education she has focussed her teaching and academic interests in cognitive behavioural approaches to care, and in teaching and learning in the practice setting.

Moyra Baldwin   is a Senior Lecturer in the Faculty of Health and Social Care at the University of Chester and is Programme Leader for the Post-graduate Certificate in Health and Social Care Commissioning. She enjoys teaching across a range of pre-registration, post-registration and postgradu-ate programmes and has been involved in education for 30 years. Her area of special interest is palliative care she has held positions that have combined practice, teaching and management. She was involved in introducing pal-liative care education at the First Moscow Hospice, Russia and facilitated seminars about palliative care in Cyprus and Holland. She has presented seminars and published on advocacy, ethics, concept analysis as a research method, and palliative care education.

Mike Burt   worked in residential care before qualifying as a social worker in 1988 following which he worked in along term children and families social work team, and in child guidance. Mike became involved in supervis-ing social work students in placement and subsequently moved to work in higher education as the programme leader for the Diploma in Social Work at Warrington Collegiate Institute in 2000. When the University of Chester incorporated the Institute's higher education in its provision Mike became Deputy Head of Social Work and was involved in the expansion of social work pre and post qualifying education and training provision. He is study-ing for a PhD in the history of social work as an occupation and has published articles about the subject.

Doreen Collyer   is a Senior Lecturer in Child Health. She has a back-ground in neonatal and children's critical care nursing and these interests form the focus of her teaching and academic work.

Julie Dulson   is a Senior Lecturer and programme leader for the pre-registration mental health programme at the University of Chester. She has a keen interest in developing service user involvement within healthcare education and has previously written and presented on this subject. Her other main research interest is the role and function of psychiatric acute inpatient wards and she previously worked on the "Search for Acute Solutions" research project with Sainsbury's Centre for Mental Health to establish ways of improving mental health acute inpatient care.

Jan Gidman's clinical background is predominately in surgical and orthopaedic nursing. She then moved into a teaching role in a large NHS Trust, before entering Higher Education ten years ago. Within her current role, Jan is responsible for the Master of Professional Education programme which is accessed by staff from both academic and practice settings in health and social care.

Jan's research interests relate to professional education and she has regularly presented at conferences and has published a number of papers and book chapters in this field. She has recently completed a research project relating to student support and is currently writing up her PhD thesis on how students learn from service users in practice settings.

Joanne Greenwood is a Senior Lecturer at the University of Chester. She has previously help senior nursing posts at various hospitals. Her nursing experience has included medicine, surgery, care of older people and Trust-wide positions. Her academic interests include ethics, evidence-based practice, and personal and professional development.

Sue Grumley trained at the Royal Liverpool Hospital College from 1979-1982 and has worked within the NHS since qualification. Her clinical interest lies within the fields of Care of the Elderly and Neurology. Her current role involves both managerial and clinical aspects allowing her to continue to develop clinically whilst being involved with shaping and developing the service provided to the service users.

Pete Hinman has 18 years post registration patient management experience in Orthopaedics, Cardiac Care, General Surgery and Accident and Emergency care. His current role as Orthopaedic Nurse Practitioner encompasses specialist clinical management of emergency orthopaedic patients throughout the admission and peri-operative pathway. Previous academic experience included clinical skills teaching, facilitating students on undergraduate and post graduate programmes and he retains an enthusiastic commitment to inter-professional collaboration along with teaching and practice development.

Neil Hosker's career in nursing started in the early 1980s. Since qualifying as a registered nurse he has worked in various nursing and senior management roles in the NHS for mental health, community and acute trusts. In 2005 he became a senior lecturer at the University of Chester teaching on the pre-registration nursing programme. His professional interests include clinical skills development, development of e-learning and online teaching materials and the use of technology by health care staff.

Formally a full time intensive care nurse, **Adam Keen** is currently working as a Senior Lecturer within the University of Chester, Faculty of Health & Social Care. His current teaching interests relate to the acute and critical care and education, including advanced resuscitation training. His research and publishing interests include critical care, information systems, dehumanisation and writing for publication. Adam has recently commenced a PhD programme.

Tom Mason has worked in mental health services in the UK, predominantly but not exclusively, for over thirty years. He has spent the last 17 years in academic posts engaging in research and publications. He was awarded an International Achievement Award in 1999 for research carried out in the forensic services of the UK and continues to be active in developing services for people with mental health problems and learning disabilities who interface with the law. Tom has published over 70 journal articles, the majority being research papers in peer reviewed journals and covers a wide range of topics. He has also co-authored and co-edited 14 books. He is currently Professor/Head of Mental Health and Learning Disabilities at the University of Chester.

Annette McIntosh is Associate Dean, Learning and Teaching, in the Faculty of Health and Social Care, University of Chester. She held various posts as a nurse, predominantly in the area of critical care, and midwife prior to entering academia. Her years in health and social care education to date have been spent in a range of roles, including clinical teacher, lecturer and principal lecturer, programme leader and quality advisor. Annette's current role involves ensuring and enhancing the quality of all learning and teaching activity, including staff development, and leading on quality reviews. Her main teaching responsibilities are lecturing on the MEd programme and supervision of Masters and PhD students. Annette's research interests encompass all aspects of teaching, learning and curriculum development, alongside an ongoing interest in sleep promotion. She is currently researching perceptions of student support.

Joy Parkes   is a Senior Lecturer in the Faculty of Health and Social Care of the University of Chester. She has special responsibility for practice learning in pre-registration adult nursing, and has been instrumental in developing criterion–based assessment of practice skills. Her practice and academic interest is in complementary and holistic therapies.

Sue Phillips   worked as a health visitor and field work teacher for many years. Her caseloads were mainly in deprived areas, with all the associated social and health problems. Following her decision to move into education, she worked for 3 years as a lecturer/practitioner, and then moved to University of Chester as a senior lecturer. She has been programme leader for both undergraduate and postgraduate programmes, and her teaching interests include public health, ethics, APEL and work based learning. She also works as an Associate Lecturer for the Open University.

Ruth Sadik   is a Senior Lecture in child health and has extensive knowledge and experience in the field gained over almost four decades.

Mike Thomas   is the Dean of the Faculty of Health and Social Care and is an experienced clinician and educator, having worked within a variety of settings. He is responsible for the strategic and operational management of the Faculty of Health and Social Care within the University of Chester and has membership of University Executive Group. Mike served as a submariner and radio operator for several years within the Royal Navy before entering the nursing profession.

Whilst working in Leeds, Mike became involved with the deployment of education resettlement of military service leavers and for five years has been working on a project to enhance the resettlement of medically discharged personnel from the tri-Services. Mike's role within the education resettlement project is that of strategic lead for the assessment and effective placement of medically discharged personnel.

Mike has worked as both a mental health clinician and an educationalist for twenty five years. He is a trustee of three charities.

Mike has published and presented papers annually since 1986 and has written chapters in books ranging from patient assessment, sexual health, professional issues and cognitive behavioural psychotherapy.

Jan Woodhouse   has had a long clinical career in the hospital setting. Since moving into higher education she has taken a focus on palliative care, the teaching of research, and education. She had edited *Strategies for*

Healthcare: How to Teach in the 21st Century, a book on evidence-based teaching strategies and is currently co-editing another book on key concepts in palliative care.

Jan has an interest in the use of the humanities in health care, which has taken a focus on storytelling, narratives and art therapy. Consequently she is helping to set up a programme of study in art therapy. The interest in art has helped in her academic studies as she is currently a PhD student looking at the topic of 'Personal grooming'.

Introduction

Jill McCarthy and Pat Rose

This book seeks to address the question: is evidence-based practice best practice? It was conceived at a staff conference at the University of Chester where we, the editors, are employed. In his introduction to the conference, the Dean of Faculty of Health and Social Care, Professor Mike Thomas (lead author of Chapter 1) discussed a burgeoning interest in values-based care as an adjunct to evidence-based practice. We discussed this with him over coffee and both expressed an interest in exploring this concept further. We sought the interest of colleagues and discovered this was an area which people throughout the faculty felt strongly about and many expressed an interest in contributing to a book. We asked these people to provide a more detailed idea of related issues affecting the health and social care professions. A key issue emerging was the dominance of positivist science within evidence-based practice with consequent devaluing of professional expertise and service users' values. These themes have thus become the focus of this book and vignettes have been used to illustrate the concepts discussed. The different approaches to the chapters represent the range of writing styles of the authors and thus widen the appeal of the book.

The book begins by exploring the history and politics of evidence-based practice and values. Within Chapter 1, it becomes evident that the political and social drivers inevitably led to the dominance of measurable outcomes and research-led practice. The chapter then examines the backlash against this dominance and subsequent re-emergence of humanistic values and holistic care. This provides a background to the argument posed in Chapter 2 that knowledge emerging from scientific study is only a part of evidence-based practice, the others being professional expertise and service user involvement. This chapter further examines the nature of evidence from a variety of sources and proposes complexity theory as a way of understanding the relationships between them.

Chapter 3 re-examines the notion of caring as a science and an art. Whilst caring behaviours can be seen to rely on a competent technical ability drawn from science, it is argued that the expressive elements of caring involve human relationships and values and are more closely related to the characteristics of art. This leads to questions posed in Chapter 4 about what it means to be human and focuses attention on four interrelated concepts that contribute to our humanistic concept of health and social care delivery: reductionism, holism, values and humanism.

Valuing professional judgement, a cornerstone of values-based care, is the focus of Chapter 5. Here, the nature of professional practice and professionalism are explored, as are the application of professional judgement, intuition, mentorship and patronage. To complement this discussion, the concept of respecting the values of individuals, a long-held central tenet for health and social care delivery, is examined in Chapter 6. This incorporates the notion of the expert patient, recognition of the value of diversity and the importance of the partnership between service users and health and social care professionals.

The final chapter draws together all of these themes and proposes a strategy for driving forward the values-based care agenda through pre- and postqualification education, values-based central policies and local management initiatives.

This book is aimed at students in the field of health and social care undertaking modules in evidence-based practice, ethics or research at undergraduate and postgraduate levels. It will also be of value to health and social care practitioners, managers, commissioners and policy makers as they strive to implement the recommendations in National Standard Frameworks to provide both evidence-based interventions and a humanistic approach to service users. Whilst rooted in the United Kingdom's approach to health and social care delivery, the ideas proposed in this book will be of value to practitioners in societies where similar issues are being raised.

The application of values-based care within practice contexts is brought to life through vignettes describing the experience of practitioners and service users. This bridges the gap between the sometimes complex theoretical discussion and the real world of health and social care practice.

1 The Emergence of Evidence-Based Practice

Mike Thomas, Mike Burt and Joy Parkes

Evidence-based practice (EBP) is currently the dominant model of health care intervention in the United Kingdom. As it values measurement and quantification, it has gained this status in a relatively short space of time, helped by a number of political, managerial and philosophical drivers emerging in separate arenas. EBP is not, however, new and has been the driving force within the quantitative science paradigm throughout its historical development and could be viewed as the bulwark in its battle with the developments of social conflict theory and the popularity of qualitative research methodologies within the social sciences.

The adoption by the medical profession of EBP and its subsequent support by the Cochrane Collaboration (a not-for-profit organisation supporting the practice and dissemination of systematic reviews in health care) may be seen as its entry into the modern context of health care, and its use is now widespread in all practice-based health professions. Its central tenets are that all health care interventions should be based on best evidence, which may be local, and based upon action research, and that it should be effective, particularly in comparison to other interventions. Effectiveness (achievement of desired outcome), alongside efficiency (productive with the minimum of waste or effort), meets one of two governmental requirements for public spending on care, and central support for EBP can be seen in the introduction of the National Institute for Clinical Excellence (NICE), now known as the National Institute for Health and Clinical Excellence.

The medical profession prides itself on its objective, scientific past, although this may not always be observed in clinical practice. Philosophy may be said to have as much of a claim to the truth as any science. A reflection upon one's own values, followed by exploration, discovery and confirmation may be seen as equally important; a final knowledge of those values adding to the efficiency of the practitioner. The training of potential medical staff involves the study of physical sciences. It was not too arduous for the profession to apply the concept of effectiveness to quantitative approaches such as data collection, particularly when the Cochrane Collaboration produced systematic reviews on available published data alongside guidelines produced by NICE regarding the introduction of new interventions.

It is interesting to note that, in the UK publicly funded health system, effectiveness is allied to cost. Thomas (2008) observed that effective, widely applicable interventions reduce service user symptoms and poor health, resulting in an important behavioural change – namely, the service user requires less public-funded intervention. Thus, intervention that is cost-effective is also viewed as efficient. There is a value placed on effectiveness and efficiency that places a moral obligation on modern health care practitioners, and reflective conversation is at the heart of a commitment to improve practice. It is proposed that, in essence, the health and social care practitioner has a moral responsibility to provide effective and efficient interventions. This is supported by Holm (2004), who also notes that EBP attempts to control health and social care costs, imposing a moral obligation on practitioners to provide evidence that any intervention used is effective.

Evidence-based practice provides a rationale for politicians and policy makers to gain some control over spending. The argument that EBP also allows practitioners to abandon ineffective interventions and introduce better models allowing politicians to manage a finite financial budget may appear hollow during a so-called credit crunch when billions of pounds may be found to bail out large financial institutions. EBP, in effect, has to formalise both the preferred quantitative approach of the last 20 years alongside a wider acceptance of qualitative approaches, providing a clearer impression of what service users need, together with what they increasingly want.

EBP does allow different health and social care practitioners to explore and study interventions from their own practice standpoint. Medicine, according to Sackett et al. (2000), employs evidence-based approaches because it allows the practitioner to use diagnostic treatment and rehabilitative regimes that have themselves been rigorously examined. Medical practitioners can have the confidence in their own clinical skills to balance the risks and benefits of different interventions, reaching a judgement on which course of action to take whilst taking into account the service user's concerns and expectations.

A doctor may find a fair proportion of any accessed data to be quantitative and the same model espoused by Sackett et al. (2000) could be used by a health professional or by a social care professional accessing data that is more qualitative by design and content. This is understandable given the biological determinism found in the curriculum of medical and health sciences education, compared with the social construct focus dominant in the curriculums of other professions such as social work. Yet the central core of EBP is its emphasis on good, solid research which demonstrates the effectiveness and efficiency of interventions and, importantly, attempts to retain the service user and carer views of intervention itself, the so-called acceptability principle. This individual perspective can, in turn, provide some defence against a generalised approach to evidence-based studies.

The use of EBP has spread since the early 1990s and is now firmly established, an achievement worthy of mention. It is not often that a movement gains such widespread acceptance in such a short time frame across so many health and social care professions, policy makers, sections of academia and the government as budget holder. The welfare state as a publicly funded structure has existed for more than 60 years, but proponents of EBP, whilst claiming a response to the culture of hearsay practice, have made no claims that, prior to its adoption, the nation's health care was based on invalid or unreliable data as illustrated in Vignette 1.1. They have however come close with the insistence that EBP does lead to a cessation of inappropriate invalid practices.

Vignette 1.1

My doctor always used to tell me to go to bed and lie flat when I had lumbago. Now, he calls it back pain and he has sent me on a course where they tell me to take pain killers and keep as mobile as possible. How come it can suddenly change like this? I used to enjoy my week in bed with my wife fussing over me – it brought us closer.

The Political Context of EBP

To understand its adoption, EBP must be contextualised within a historical perspective involving political, philosophical and managerial developments. In medicine, the resurgence of biological determinism coincided with the political and managerial focus of controlling public funding alongside the rise of entrepreneurship as the new business theory. For other health and social care professions, the rise of consumer power, of advocacy and internet groups and of the independent sector has impacted on service users' claims for more autonomy and control over their own care.

With the change of focus, the NHS altered beyond recognition from its roots in social welfare. Long-term care moved to the fee-charging private companies now termed independent care providers from the District General Hospitals. The Ambulance Service and the primary care providers converted to semi-independent NHS Trusts, the 1990 NHS and Community Care Act requiring Trusts to behave like businesses and be active in the marketplace. This social engineering became clear a year later when, in 1991, the NHS was again restructured to encourage the invention of a new internal market. Regional Health Authorities were re-designated Commissioners and instructed to purchase health care from the provider Trusts now selling their services. Both parties formalised these arrangements through contracts, although such contracts have no real basis in contract law, thus demonstrating the centrally controlled power held by government. The Department of Health, however, ensured commitments made in these contracts must be honoured.

Effectiveness and efficiency, originally measured through the provision of local services to meet local targets, now faced a fundamentally different measurement. Provision of service had still to be focused on local needs, but annual budgets were abandoned. Trusts were instructed to both generate their own income and to compete against other local services, particularly through the strategy of undercutting each other, an added benefit being the reduction of centrally allocated funds. This was at a time when EBP was beginning to gain a voice, and the political imperative for the new market was increasing efficiency and user choice.

Talbot-Smith and Pollock (2006) highlight the fact that the previously held local pride in building a hospital was now dead. Between 1990 and 1994, 254 hospitals were closed in England and Wales. During these years, the government introduced a new tier of resource-intensive service into the health sector. Trusts desperate to avoid closure spent more and more funding on contract management, competing for the tender of risk management and financial services. To add to their problems, the government used the 1990 Act to allow private profit-based companies to hold contracts to deliver estates, capital management and technological provision. These were to be paid not from what had previously been a Department of Health service (regional offices being closed), but from the Trust budgets. As Talbot-Smith and Pollock (2006) observe, the Trusts were now trading in the newly invented health market, selling their services to service brokers (Commissioners) and, in turn, buying consultancy services to keep their organisation competitive against other market players including other parts of the NHS.

This competition forced some out of the market and the merging of others. This removed the financial burden on central government. Local services, particularly capital estates, expanded to take on the extra services now being offered from a smaller number of NHS Trusts. Private, independent, profit-orientated companies were allowed to form a partnership with Trusts to erect new buildings, expand existing estates and operate the services such as maintenance and cleaning in these buildings and, in some cases, share rental leases for retail outlets. Much like a mortgage or long-term loan, the profit-based partner would be paid for their contribution, the Trust paying them over a long period of time, guaranteeing income in excess of 25 years in most cases. As we have seen, over 250 hospitals closed in the three years of the new market and by 2005 only 50 hospitals had increased their building or estate; 42 of these were held in Private Finance Initiative contracts (Talbot-Smith and Pollock, 2006).

Since the turn of the century, the primary care sector has been assimilated into the current Primary Care Trusts (PCTs) and the effectiveness and efficiency focused on preventative and community care. Government targets are aimed at reducing cancers, strokes, cardiopulmonary problems, simultaneously transferring much of the care for chronic and long-term conditions into the community. Consequently, Primary Care Trusts have recently been split into two services, one a commissioning arm buying services from providers and the other the provider arm. The old District General Hospitals which evolved into NHS secondary and tertiary Care Trusts have undergone yet another change; several of them are now designated Foundation Trusts with even more independence from central control. Via a tendering process, they can compete for the delivery of services against local PCT providers, independent organisations and the voluntary sector and can purchase other sites in order to expand services.

The system is now embedded in contract law, and there are a number of regulatory bodies which oversee quality and provide guidance on provision, tendering, Foundation status and local requirements. The PCT commissioners in turn base their decisions regarding tendering on efficiency (cost), effectiveness (achievement of outcomes) and acceptability by the local population.

Compared to the closure of the great industrial bases in the UK, such a radical dismantling of a centrally funded National Health Service occurred with little social unrest, with managerial enthusiasm in a majority of cases, and all in the last 20 years. When presented against the privatisation of the health system and the need to operate within highly controlled budgets, the impact of evidence-based practice is, politically, not too surprising. A political lead was taken on adopting such a system as EBP, its attractiveness to the political leaders self-evident. It removes ineffective interventions, introduces new, more effective care allied to efficiency and it has a strong element, linked to action research, of the user's perspective in its philosophy. The science of health care delivery via EBP was promulgated at just the right time to meet government expectations. It also lent credibility to the decision-making of managers, providing a rationale for discussions with contract holders who, in turn, had been through a socio-cultural change.

EBP in Social Work

The tension between evidence and values-based approaches has featured in the development of the social care and social work knowledge base since the mid-Victorian period. The Charity Organisation Society was formed in 1869 to provide an alternative to indiscriminate charitable giving, attaching importance to what they regarded as a scientific approach to distributing charity. Their casework approach thoroughly examined the individual circumstances of applicants, and determined how specific provision might be successfully used by the recipient (Woodroofe, 1961).

The development of knowledge from surveys of the poor, the impact of economic cycles and the social sciences reduced the significance attached to individual culpability, informing the development of a much wider range of provision. Harris (1999: 48), from the beginning the 20th century, argues that 'one of the most striking features of "social reform" literature over the next 30 years was to be the continuing interaction between sociological theory, social philosophy, empirical investigation, casework, and the analysis of practical social policy'. She highlights in the development of this social-scientific culture, the role of the Fabian Society, local Charity Organisation Societies, and, subsequently, the British Institute of Social Service, the Guild of Help movement, and the councils of social welfare and civic trusts of the Edwardian period. Harris (1999) argues that the development of social welfare provision was influenced by the social philosophy of the Idealists, and notes, in particular, the role of Edward Urwick. He was the first head of the Charity Organisation Society's School of Sociology in 1903 and, subsequently, the first head of the department of social science and administration at the London School of Economics in 1912. Harris suggests that, after the Victorian and Edwardian periods, social scientists became increasingly aware of the limitations of biological and natural-scientific models. Idealist academics and philosophers were involved in establishing early departments of social science where the first academically trained social workers and social scientists were taught. She further suggests that Idealism didn't discourage the empirical research of specific social problems, but claimed that the facts were meaningless without a broader vision and framework for the reconstruction of the whole of society within which the moral character of individuals could be reformed.

This framework promoted the creation of a state based on the contribution of individuals, including the poor, as responsible citizens to society.

The application of social science knowledge to individual cases within the social casework of the period was formulated by Richmond's (1917) influential *Social Diagnosis*, written explicitly in the USA to assert that social work could be regarded as a profession. She wrote about the systematic collection of social evidence, drawing inferences, developing hypotheses and making interpretations. Clement Brown (1939) identifies this tradition in social casework in the UK, also drawing attention to the different role of a social worker who emphasises the importance of a continuing relationship with a service user through which change is effected, itself a role developed in the USA and influenced by psychoanalytic theory.

Following post-war legislation, social work roles developed within state provision. The journals of the different occupational groups contained articles which were based on empirical research and used to promote a particular development for policy and practice. However, the range of material was sufficiently limited to the extent that very little academic research had been carried out in the UK. The National Institute for Social Work Training, established in 1961, included a centre for research. The Seebohm Report (1968) advocated that social service departments should be established, recommending that more research should be carried out within these. The influence of the study of sociology in the 1960s enhanced social workers' understanding of the family, but also led to a radical critique of the casework method which was perceived to locate problems within individuals. This radical critique argued that the problems which disadvantaged people experienced arose from the structural inequalities of society, and that they should be addressed at that level. Social service departments established a research function when they were created in 1971 and the Department of Health set up the Personal Social Services Council, an independent advisory, research and development body.

The effectiveness of social work became an important issue in the 1970s. Goldberg and Fruin (1976) pointed out that some social workers took the view that research and social work practice were not compatible because of the uniqueness of individuals and that a therapeutic relationship could not be scientifically analysed. They suggested that social workers sometimes resisted the clarification of goals in their work. In her summary of social work research, Crousaz (1981) points out that evaluative research was very limited in social work, the size and design of studies failing to meet the requirements of rigorous experimental methods. She argued: 'If evaluation is to go further than a limited measure of success or failure according to the criteria set up, there must be some attempt to isolate the factors which might contribute to success or failure … It may in fact be just those aspects of the relationship which are most unconscious and hardest to articulate and categorise: empathy, caring, or a social worker's own personality and adjustment which are the key features. Or it may be aspects of the client not generally measured, such as motivation to change' (Crousaz, 1981: 37).

The 1980s saw the continued advancement of evidence-based and values-based approaches as alternative knowledge bases for the development of effective practice. Sheldon (1986: 240) argued for 'the fostering of a greater respect for empiricism; for putting behind us our tendency to practice or to teach on the basis of ideas that we happen to find congenial, rather than those which have stood up to practical test'. He draws attention to the predominance of the casework method in studies, mainly from the USA, up to 1972 which failed to show the effectiveness of social work practice. He contrasts these with studies from 1973 onwards, again primarily from the USA, which were more specific in focus, used smaller samples and in which social workers made more direct interventions in behavioural problems. Sheldon quotes Fischer (1985) who suggested that by 1973 there had been a failure to demonstrate that systematic improvements could be made, beyond the natural power of the environment or the passage of time, to a wide range of problems encountered by service users, but that we certainly knew about values!

Along with other professions, the use of the specific term 'evidence-based practice' started to be used within social work during the 1990s. Webb (2001) suggests that the article by Macdonald and Sheldon (1992), 'Contemporary studies of the effectiveness of social work', prepared the way the way for evidence-based practice in the 1990s. Webb offers a detailed critique of the attempt to apply an evidence-based practice approach to all decisions, questioning whether scientific approaches to behaviour were themselves able to provide the evidence that they could be made to work. He expresses concern that although the use of research evidence in practice in itself is not problematic, the assumptions of evidence-based practice as a methodology for practice itself are too limiting in enabling practitioners to respond to the range of situations they face in practice. He further states that it feeds the managerial agenda and because the basis of the approach is in behaviourism and positivism, it is flawed. It assumes that a rational agent is in a position throughout their work to apply obvious conclusions from findings to logical decision making. Webb (2001: 74) suggests that 'Evidence-based practice effectiveness sits comfortably alongside the new managerialism in social work. The recent imposition of a cognitive-behavioural model in the probation service in England is a further example of this tendency to enforce standardised methods and supposedly scientific models of intervention'.

Sheldon's (2001) reply to Webb emphasises that alternative methodological approaches have not been shown to be effective in social work and are advanced because academics may favour them. He suggests that there is a great deal of evidence that behavioural approaches do work. In their review of this debate, Butler and Pugh (2004) assert that there are basic problems surrounding the assumptions made by supporters of evidence-based practice regarding the objectivity, not to mention the reliability, of observation itself, of assessing different sorts of evidence, and of the processes of inference which lead from evidence to explanation. They reject a hierarchy of methodologies which places a positivist approach at the top and subjective approaches such as narrative accounts of personal experience at the bottom. They further argue that isolating actions to be examined from their broader contexts leaves the fundamental causes of social problems unexplored, thereby attempting to depoliticise social work research and social work itself.

Gray and McDonald (2006) have questioned whether the nature of social work practice can be reduced to measurable and quantifiable data. They postulate that 'the adoption of evidence-based practice can be best understood as a continuation of long-standing attempts to deal with the ubiquity of ambiguity and uncertainty in social work' (Gray and McDonald, 2006: 12). Van de Luitgaarden (2009) argues that evidence-based practice is related to a rational choice model of decision making. He points out that scholars in the field of judgement and decision making have found this approach impractical for certain types of decision making and that it is mainly those types of tasks with which social workers are principally concerned. He points to the significance of perceptions rather than measurable factors, and of constantly changing factors in social situations.

The modernisation of social care since the advent of Labour governments from 1997 has led to an increase in various forms of support for the development of research based on the government's principal concern to identify and disseminate evidence of what works. Foremost amongst the initiatives has been the establishment of the Social Care Institute for Excellence (SCIE) in 2001. SCIE is responsible for disseminating research knowledge to the occupational sector of social care. The Joint University Council Social Work Education Committee (JUC-SWEC) has published a strategy to significantly improve the quality and quantity of social work research in higher education institutions in the UK (JUC-SWEC, 2006). The report states that a long-term strategy is required to build a research capability within social work, which has developed as an applied policy and practice discipline but with significantly less funding than is obtained by, for example, health research. The report refers to the evidence base of social work but prefers the term 'evidence-informed practice'. Within social work departments of Higher Education Institutions, research networks have become active, including Making Research Count and Research in Practice. Commensurate with policy developments which involve service users and carers in active participation in meeting their own care needs, there is an increasing involvement of service users and carers in directly carrying out research as shown in Vignette 1.2.

Vignette 1.2

My husband is in the early stages of Alzheimer's disease. Recently we were both invited to participate in a research study looking at what support needs to be in place for both me and my husband. We are both in different focus groups which explore our views from our own perspectives. My husband was a principal lecturer at a local college and he feels this will be his final opportunity to have his name on a publication and also, because he is quite well known, it will make people want to read it. For me it will be the first time my name has ever been in print and that makes me feel that what I have to say is important.

At the beginning of the new century, the current position is that there is a strongly identified need for a significant increase in the availability of research evidence to inform policy and practice in social work. However, this drive is within the context of valuing the validity of different epistemological bases. It is accepted that where there is evidence available of effective interventions, these should be used to inform the practice social workers are frequently involved in, that is in complex social situations. Consequently, social workers can be expected to be reflexive about the intentions, nature and impact of the way in which they engage with service users and carers and the dominance of EBP in healthcare has not currently made a major impact in social work. It remains to be seen whether social work will be able to resist the governmental culture which emphasises efficiency and effectiveness in financial rather than human costs.

The Management Culture

The culture of efficiency has been closely aligned to quality and the belief that quality provides a competitive edge in the marketplace providing a guide to value. In turn, value is a disjunctive concept in the sense that the word value has different meanings in different situations. Value is often used to refer to an amount, usually of money, but sometimes of goods that a person can exchange for something else. It may also refer to personal satisfaction in that the amount a person exchanges is within a given range – the 'value-for-money' feeling. It can also mean the present worth of something to gain something else. That is, the price of an object in a collector's market would have a higher value to a collector than an interested onlooker. Values may also mean moral principles. Balogun and Hailey (2004) suggest that corporate values were viewed by managers in the 1980s as a mechanism to steer organisations towards better efficiency and they were supported in this by the growth in human resource management methods which held cultural change programmes in high regard. There was a strongly held belief in the entrepreneurial spirit which was pushed by the government as not only good business technique, but also morally acceptable.

If organisations provided employees with a package of corporate values which emphasised entrepreneurialism, then the workforce would be more likely to innovate; there would be a decreased need for bureaucratic proce-dures and, in turn, a reduced interference by management. A twin belief was that organisations would be less risk-averse and more enthusiastic in taking control of their own direction. Later evidence demonstrated that such beliefs were misplaced. For example, the value statements marketed by companies, often in the form of Charters, lost their currency when it became apparent that senior managers were not altering their own behaviours, and the more alert workers disseminated a sense of cynicism when they perceived that management were manipulating the staff. There was also an inbuilt mech-anism for undermining the value-based approach when staff did embrace the belief in self-determination; as the company became more diverse in its activities, so the idea of core values became more diluted. This was especially predominant in organisations such as hospitals and services such as com-munity care. The core problems arose from the lack of commitment by senior managers to improve inter-organisational communications and the flow of information. There was also a lack of awareness of the extra work required to involve both staff and service users in the organisational values by the use of workshops, briefings, updates and so on. In the mid-1980s, there was a form of marketing and branding in the commercial world which emphasised val-ues when, in fact, they continued to practise in a profit-orientated way which rejected value-based care.

Lencioni (2002) observed that the public and employees soon saw through these managerial approaches and by the start of this century corporate values were viewed as a capitalist attempt to be politically correct. By then, a consider-able amount of damage had been done to those very workers who should have benefited from value-based objectives. The issue appeared to be one of trust between those who managed and those who were managed – ironically itself a value concept. George (2001) suggests that trust is an important organisational virtue because mutual trust between staff increases efficiency, whereas a lack of trust decreases creativity and increases control over the work environment which leads to loss of profitability. It is interesting that the concept of trust has such a hold in the for-profit business community as trust itself can have different uses in different contexts. At its basic level, trust involves giving to another that which one holds valuable (money, knowledge freedom, information, consent or secrets) and feeling emotionally secure that what is given is safe with the other. Yet Joni (2004) suggests that there is also a professional trust and a structural trust. In the professional context, trust is based on the individuals' knowledge or ability in their field of expertise and their capability to provide informed, disinterested, objective and truthful advice whilst structural trust is based on the roles and responsibilities given to an individual, for example a doctor, nurse, police officer or faith minister, by others either in their contract of employment, by the law or by cultural norms.

A further blow to the customer-first philosophy had been the government's attempts to restore trust in business practices by its insistence on accountability, transparency and public involvement. O'Neill (2002) suggested that the drive for accountability merely led to an increase in bureaucracy, burdening public institutions with increased costs.

Public service organisations have been encouraged by politicians to structure themselves in a market-orientated way so that the capitalist drive for efficiency and effectiveness has an impact on public spending itself. The new emphasis on customer satisfaction at this time was fortuitous. It meant a closer relationship, superficially at least, between public-funded bodies and the ethos of the market; both accepted the ideology of social and moral responsibilities, both claimed to meet customer needs and provide good services and both accepted the inclusion of interest groups in their strategic planning.

The dynamism of the free market was viewed as an important catalyst to change in the moribund health and social care system in the UK. The simultaneous growth of evidence-based practice in the public services reflected the emphasis on efficiency and effectiveness which motivated the drive to increase profits in the business sector. In many ways, the evidence-based care model is a capitalist device with the added value of being ethically acceptable. It was, therefore, very timely and welcomed in different areas: by the medical profession because of its science-based results; by managers because it provided socially acceptable rationales for health and social care strategies; by auditors because it provided comparative measurements and league tables; by commercial companies because it provided a selling angle and by politicians because it provided possible reductions in public spending. Overall, evidence-based practice can be seen as good value for money. There has, however, been little, if any, detailed consideration of the nature of these values themselves and whether the concept of value is commensurate with business practices and evidence-based care.

Values-based Care

The concept of values-based care has been gaining ground within health and social care services over the last decade. This holistic form of care has already been implemented within some areas of mental health services and community services (Olsen, 2000) due, it can be reasoned, to unease with over-reliance on evidence-based practice. Values-based care is a blending of the values of both the service user and the health and social care professional, thus creating a true, as opposed to a tokenistic, partnership. It is suggested that the importance of values in care may have been overlooked because they are presumed to be shared unless clearly openly conflicting (Olsen, 2000). The Royal College of General Practitioners (RCGP, 2007: statement 1) recommends in their core RCGP curriculum, that all general practitioners should be able to 'understand the nature of values and how these impact on healthcare' and 'recognise their personal values and how these effect their decision-making'. Thus, the importance of values-based care for this group of professionals is clearly stated.

NHS Education for Scotland (2008), which as a country may be considered to be driving the UK move towards values-based care (see, for example, Mental Health (Care and Treatment) (Scotland) Act 2003), published a list of values according to three staff groups, a selection of which are listed here:

Delegates at a conference regarding mental health recovery

- Core beliefs
- Principles – cultural, individual
- Anything that's valued
- Social values
- Valuing neighbours
- Your perspective on the world.

Managers/Chief executives

- Right and wrong
- Belief systems
- Ideals and priorities
- Things that govern behaviour and decisions
- Conscience.

Trainee psychiatrists

- What you believe in
- Principles
- Personal motivating force
- Primary reference points.

As can be seen, these are broad headings which encompass multiple ideas and personal philosophies. Values-based care cannot be fitted into neat pigeon holes, nor can professionals be given a simple 'how to' manual. This model of care leans heavily on the professionalism of the health and social care worker gained through knowledge, experience and respect for service users' views. Little (2002: 319) when discussing healthcare stated that 'If we are to seek a new model for a reconstructed view of health care, the term "values-based medicine" might have more power and relevance than "humanistic medicine"'. Health care provision cannot be separated from universal values such as caring and compassion and thus consideration of individual values cannot be ignored, especially when these are in opposition to evidence-based practice (Olsen, 2000), as illustrated in some of the vignettes contained within this book.

The Nature of Values

As previously noted, the concept of value can mean different things to different people, depending on the context in which it is applied. In general, however, a value is likely to be based on the desirability of acquisition in terms of its immediate or potential practical benefits, for example toothpaste as immediate and stocks or shares as potential benefits. The price of such objects is determined in monetary terms – a different type of value in that the cost of something will depend on its accessibility and whether the buyer feels the cost is a fair exchange and value for money. This model has been increasingly applied to health and social care because value in economic terms can be measured in both mathematical quantities (the amount of money, materials and resources) and customer satisfaction, whilst personal health and social circumstances (well-being) can be viewed as a valuable asset. This model easily absorbs scientific approaches of evidence-based practice. Evidence-based care can provide an additional evaluation to its therapeutic value by embracing the economic concept of value, thereby making comparisons based on efficiency and effectiveness. Such perceptions of value, whilst deeply ingrained in society, are based on whether something is perceived as desirable or not. However, despite repeated attempts by economists to forge a link between for-profit capitalist value and ethics, the concept of values as moral principles remains elusive in the economic market. As moral principles, values provide guidelines for individual and societal actions and, additionally, can be ascribed to the regard one person has for another – their integrity, trustworthiness and moral character. These two definitions of value can often be opposed when related to those characterisations and actions which individuals undertake in the pursuit of profit. Here, the stress is less on what is valuable and more on subjectivity in the context of personal judgements based on moral acceptability. A classic example is the debate which surrounded HIV vaccinations, and whether pharmaceutical companies should provide lower-cost products to economically poor countries. The companies initially took the view that their investments required a profit return. Only after they accepted that such a stance reflected poorly on their organisational values did they start to provide cheaper products, and only after action groups had lobbied for values as moral principles rather than monetary gain.

Robinson (2001) discusses value judgements in terms of a prioritisation model in which an individual gauges the importance of personal values through a form of cognitive filtering, citing Raths et al. (1978) who proposed that an individual examines choice, worth and behaviour in order to prioritise values. Choice involves freedom to choose, an environment providing comparative choices and a consideration of the consequences of the choice made. Worth involves examining the desirability and contentment provided by whatever one chooses to value and articulating and affirming that choice in the public domain. Behaviours include the application of a chosen personal value to one's life and applying it repeatedly. One of the important consequences to consider is the impact of a chosen value on others close to oneself and on society generally. The conflict of holding a personal moral value which conflicts with a generally held societal value can lead to moral dissonance. Examples may include a politician who, believing in peace through dialogue, may have to present a public face of supporting military intervention in order to protect their own career, or a minister of faith having to defend scriptural teaching during social unrest, or the situation described in Vignette 1.3.

Vignette 1.3

As a Health Visitor I remember calling on one family who were struggling with child-rearing. We had discussed smacking in the past and the mother felt that as it had never done her any harm she felt it was a good way of teaching her child right from wrong. Despite all my explanations, and my strong belief that smacking is wrong, during this visit I had to watch silently as she smacked her three-year-old child when he pestered her for attention because smacking is not illegal and society generally supports it.

John Locke (1974) examined the confusion surrounding concepts when a complex idea such as a value is reduced to too many simple ideas, famously giving the example of not assuming that just because an animal has spots it must be a leopard. He argued that words and their definitions not only lead to a taxonomical order, but also help the individual avoid confusion. Words aid a person by making clear the distinction between things, and the similarities and differences between things that appear on the surface to be the same. Some ideas, however, are simple and others more complex. Locke (1632–1704) suggested that simple concrete concepts are archetypes, and a visual presentation will often succeed in getting everyone generally to accept the idea – a chair, for instance, can be seen as an archetypical concept. More complex concepts require the relationships between ideas to be made clear. For instance, a car is an archetypical concept in the modern world but, as there are different types of cars and different models, the archetype becomes more complex. Another layer would be transport where the idea of car would also have a relationship with train, bus and plane. But if an idea is used outside its context, or replicates existing words with different meanings, it loses substance. It becomes an inadequate method of conveying ideas because it causes confusion. The use of the word value in both moral and commercial contexts, and the inter-weaving of meanings in different settings, may have provided an intellectual device to merge public funded health and social care with for-profit organisations. Reinforcing this view, Smith (1929) states that Kant (1724–1804) takes a slightly different approach to Locke, suggesting instead that judgements can be made based on both ideas and ideals. Both have the power to provide a practical basis for actions and, therefore, act as regulatory principles for a person's behaviour. Moral concepts, however, do not necessarily rest on reasoning alone, but also on the pleasure (or displeasure) of the consequences of actions. Kant argued that some ideas appear complex, but are actually archetypes, suggesting, for example, that virtue and wisdom can be seen as moral values but can equally be viewed as regulatory principles. This is because, when related to rules of law or cultural behaviours, they provide boundaries, preventing completely free actions. Kant would accept that no individual fully achieves a wise and virtuous life. This ideal acts as an archetype because it can be used as a comparative social model, placing values on socially accepted ideas and behaviours. Even though such concepts have no objective reality, they nevertheless constitute an idea in the mind which allows the individual to evaluate moral worth and make a value judgement. The attainment of an ideal is, for Kant, unrealistic and so we allocate value to the value concepts themselves and these values act as archetypes for personal behaviour and actions.

Mautner (1997) defines another perception of values. He writes in his dictionary that some actions can be value-free, especially in empirical science, because research alone does not establish whether some thing, or some action or some state is good or bad. These are value-neutral until someone provides a value judgement to the results. Scientific enquiry can provide causes and effects, predictions and explanations, but not value judgements. This argument has some exponents but research does not occur in a vacuum. Inevitably, it must have value judgements and applicability placed on its results; the concept of value-free research is not widely accepted.

Robinson (2001) sees some difficulties with Raths et al.'s (1978) model and its roots in Kantian's regulatory principles. He asks who, for instance, defines a value as socially desirable and whether a model based on reasoning makes assumptions that an individual is both rational and able to make choices. Even then, there are potential clashes seen in the periodic requests from service users and families to be given medication or therapies that are deemed too expensive by regulatory bodies. Even when the majority recognise the reasoning behind such efficiency arguments, the value judgements can alter when faced with the individual or a loved one who is affected. Those with power and authority will want to impose the values of the majority for cost-effective care, but the individual practitioner may want to impose a moral principle of valuing individuals. Illness and poor social circumstances can also affect choice and decision making and the articulation of moral choices can be difficult in emotional environments. Robinson thus questions how an individual can demonstrate moral values if personal values are left outside the working environment.

Robinson et al. (2003) stress that value prioritisation requires a degree of reflective skills and the opportunity to explore values with others to ascertain the consequences of one's choices and any possible future responses to moral actions. In other words, value judgement is a learned ability and does not occur spontaneously or independently. Edwards (1998) suggests that this learning itself occurs in a relational and complex environment where those that provide moral guidance or judgements are themselves morally judged. In the context of positivist research, the investigator is required to leave their own values and ideals outside the research paradigm itself, an apparently contradictory stance unless the research is then subjected to value-judgements by external referees acting as guides to the research method's reliability.

Russell (1961) takes the historical view, discussing Hegel's (1770–1831) stance which supports Robinson et al.'s (2003) view, that the ultimate imposition of moral authority is given by the state. The issue of social power, therefore, cannot be disengaged from the consequences of value choices. Most democratic governments manage a benign form of authority in such areas by condoning organisations that are not deemed harmful to the common good, allowing interest and pressure groups a certain amount of independence. This political philosophy is an adequate framework to support differing social interests, and its basis in law and rationality allows health care practitioners to hold and practise particular aspirational values of their own. In health and social care settings, the complexity approach (discussed in detail in Chapter 2) provides a rationale for the inclusivity of users, carers and workers, supporting the case for valuing user involvement in service delivery. This is because an individual can represent a group interest, and is therefore a means to reach aspirational ethical values which have a relationship with corporate and political values. By including user representatives in strategic and operational issues, it can be argued that the voice of the community is heard, irrespective of whether individuals bring their own or their constituents' values to the organisation.

EBP can be viewed as an historical movement arising from the medical profession's response to governmental targets regarding health and social well-being. The political stress on efficiency and effectiveness around public spending provides an environment within which a more explicit numerically transparent method of data collection and analysis can flourish. Alongside the political movement ran business and corporate changes in the commercial sector. These focused on organisational values in an attempt to brand products and services as desirable to service users. A synergy between the medical philosophy of learning and practice, political aspirations and commercial exploitation has thus been achieved.

The pendulum, however, may have swung too far towards the 'evidence' for efficiency and effectiveness at the expense of acceptability by health and social care users. EBP has a distinct and robust basis in clinical practice. Its values differ from political and managerial values. Nevertheless, the combination of clinical, evidence-based care, political interference and commercial profits has led to positional aspirations with health and social care services grouped into value-laden league tables.

However, the policy papers that have circulated since the NHS Next Stage Review (DH, 2008a) indicate that the pendulum may need to swing back towards a user and staff acceptability value system. There is more emphasis on the quality spectrum regarding care, although this remains within the boundaries of effectiveness and efficiency. Nursing and midwifery care, for example, is to be audited on its compassion, safety and effectiveness (DH, 2008b; Griffiths et al., 2008; Maben and Griffiths, 2008). Evidence will be accepted using both a quantitative and qualitative methodology with the open admission that the quality of care provided has failed to receive due recognition when compared to competing productivity targets. The new aspects to be measured include treatable conditions, falls, hospital-acquired infections, communication with care providers, medical administrative errors, staffing levels, well-being and satisfaction measurements. The rigour of the data indicators will be overseen by the National Quality Forum which will expect scientifically sound and usable data to demonstrate an impact on service users and national goals. Evidence-based practice is one strong area but equally there will be an expectation that new quality measures will be utilised to demonstrate the impact of care.

The Allied Health Professions (AHP) (DH, 2008c) have also agreed to develop a set of quality matrices, and will monitor personal health budgets with an emphasis on user control, choice and empowerment. The leaders of the AHP specialties are also asked to understand the realities of working in user-led, but still evidence-based and contestable, systems (McMahon, 2008).

For staff development, the government has continued to stress evidence-based practice (DH, 2008d: 36) as an 'analytical function for workforce supply and demand modelling and providing a single evidence base for the health and social care systems'. It also signals a move towards value-based care, encouraging and promoting the use of feedback from users and the public in the design of training and education of the workforce. The NHS Next Stage Review (DH, 2008d) stresses the requirement for health and social care delivery to have a culture which values staff and lifelong services alongside user, carer and public involvement. It must also make use of EBP as a means to provide evidence for the need for clinical services, and as an economic model to measure workforce effectiveness.

Evidence-based practice has also spread to the independent sector. The National Council for Voluntary Organisations (NCVO, 2007) is committed to producing a national research centre. Amongst several key principles will be the involvement of stakeholders in research activities and the development of an evidence-based culture. The research centre will also have an interest in evidence for the values, outcomes and effectiveness of service delivery.

Evidence-based practice is now a reality for the planning and delivery of health and social care in the UK. It is gaining ground in related fields such as education and environmental well-being (United Kingdom Public Health Association, 2007). It provides a robust, reliable and valid methodology underpinning a rationale for adopting values such as effectiveness, efficiency and acceptability. In certain areas – pharmacology, for example – it is the most appropriate method of data collection and analysis. In other areas, it is too susceptible to gaming where organisations play their positional aspirations by focusing on specific government performance indicators which, in reality, take resources away from overall organisational improvements.

The current trend is for more qualitative, value-based evidence to be implemented within health and social care environments in an attempt to balance the existing dominance of quantitative, evidence-based evidence and to support the inclusion of stakeholders. In the future, perhaps, reflection may be used to bridge the gap between values and action, confirming best practice whilst discovering new ways forward.

References

Balogun, J. and Hailey, V.H. (2004) *Exploring Strategic Change*. Harlow, Essex: Pearson Education Ltd.

Butler, I. and Pugh, R. (2004) 'The politics of social work research', in R. Lovelock, K. Lyons and J. Powell (eds) *Reflecting on Social Work – Discipline and Profession*. Aldershot: Ashgate, pp. 55–71.

Clement Brown, S. (1939) 'The methods of social caseworkers', in F.C. Bartlett, M. Ginsberg, E.J. Lindgreen and R.H. Thouless (eds) *The Study of Society: Methods and Problems*. London: Kegan Paul, Tench, Trubner & Co, pp. 379–401.

Crousaz, D. (1981) *Social Work: A Research Review*. London: HMSO.

Department of Health (DH) (1990) *NHS and Community Care Act*. London: Department of Health.

Department of Health (DH) (2008a) *NHS Next Stage Review – Leading Local Change*. London: Department of Health.

Department of Health (DH) (2008b) *Framing the Nursing and Midwifery Contribution – Driving up the Quality of Care*. London: Department of Health.

Department of Health (DH) (2008c) *Framing the Contribution of Allied Health Professionals – Delivering High Quality Healthcare*. London: Department of Health.

Department of Health (DH) (2008d) *High Quality Care for All – NHS Next Stage Review Final Report*. London: Department of Health.

Edwards, S.D. (ed.) (1998) *Philosophical Issues in Nursing*. London: MacMillan.

Fischer, J. (1985) Lecture and discussion at Green College, Oxford, reprinted in part in *Behavioural Social Work Review*, Spring.

George, W.W. (2001) 'Keynote Address – Academy of Management Annual Conference 2001', *Academy of Management Executives*, 15(4): 39–47.

Goldberg, E.M. and Fruin, M.J. (1976) 'Towards accountability in social work – a case review system for social workers', *British Journal of Social Work*, 6(1): 3–22.

Gray, M. and McDonald, C. (2006) 'Pursuing good practice? The limits of evidence-based practice', *Journal of Social Work*, 6(1): 7–20.

Griffiths, P., Jones, S., Maben, J. and Murrells, T. (2008) 'State of the art metrics for nursing: a rapid appraisal', *National Nursing Research Unit*. London: Kings College. Available at http://www.kcl.ac.uk/content/1/c6/04/32/19/Metricsfinalreport.pdf [accessed 29 January 2010]

Harris, J. (1999) 'Political thought and the welfare state 1870–1940: an intellectual framework for British Social Policy', in D. Gladstone (ed.) *Before Beveridge: Welfare Before the Welfare State*. London: IEA, pp. 43–63.

Holm, S. (2004) 'Evidence-based practice – the role of nursing research', in D. Tadd (ed.) *Ethical and Professional Issues in Nursing – Perspectives from Europe*. Basingstoke: Palgrave Macmillan, pp. 37–55.

Joni, S.A. (2004) 'The geography of trust', *Harvard Business Review*, March: 82–8.

JUC-SWEC (2006) *A Social Work Research Strategy in Higher Education 2006–2020*. London: Social Care Workforce Research Unit.

Lencioni, P.M. (2002) 'Make your values mean something', *Harvard Business Review*, July: 113–17.

Little, J.M. (2002) 'Humanistic medicine or values-based medicine ... what's in a name?', *Medical Journal of Australia*, 177(6): 319–21.

Locke, J. (1974) *An Essay Concerning Human Understanding*. New York: Everyman Library.

Maben, J. and Griffiths, P. (2008) 'Nursing in society: starting the debate', *National Nursing Research Unit*. London: Kings College.

MacDonald, G. and Sheldon, B. (1992) 'Contemporary studies of the effectiveness of social work', *British Journal of Social Work*, 22: 615–43.

Mautner, T. (1997) *Dictionary of Philosophy*. London: Penguin Books.

McMahon, L. (2008) 'Reading the compass – a report on a workshop event on the leadership needs of the allied health professions', *LOOP*, London: City University.

National Council for Voluntary Organisations (2007) *NCVO's Response to the OTS Consultation on a new Third Sector Research Centre – November 2007*. London: NCVO.

NHS Education for Scotland (2008) *The 10 Essential Shared Capabilities for Mental Health Practice: Learning Materials (Scotland)*. Edinburgh: NES.

Olsen, D. (2000) 'Editorial comment', *Nursing Ethics*, 7(6): 470–1.

O'Neill, O. (2002) *A Question of Trust – The BBC Reith Lectures 2002*. Cambridge: Cambridge University Press.

Raths, L., Harmin, M. and Simon, S.B. (1978) 'Values and teaching: working with values in the classroom', in S.J. Robinson (2001) *Agape – More Meaning and Pastoral Counselling*, Cardiff: Aureus Publishing, pp. 127–54.

RCGP (2007) *Being a General Practitioner*. London: RCGP. Available at: www.rcgp-curriculum.org.uk/PDF/curr_1_Curriculum_Statement_Being_a_GP.pdf [accessed 1 December 2009]

Richmond, M. (1917) *Social Diagnosis*. New York: Russell Sage Foundation.

Robinson, S.J. (2001) *Agape – More Meaning and Pastoral Counselling*. Cardiff: Aureus Publishing.

Robinson, S., Kendrick, K. and Brown, A. (2003) *Spirituality and the Practice of Health Care*. Basingstoke: Palgrave Macmillan.

Russell, B. (1961) *History of Western Philosophy*. London: Routledge.

Sackett, D.L., Strauss, S.E. and Richardson, W.S. (2000) *Evidence-based Medicine: How to Practice and Teach EBM*. London: Churchill Livingstone.

Seebohm Report (1968) *Report of the Committee on Local Authority and Allied Personal Social Services*, London: Department of Health.

Sheldon, B. (1986) 'Social work effectiveness experiments: review and implications', *British Journal of Social Work*, 16: 223–42.

Sheldon, B. (2001) 'The validity of evidence-based practice in social work: a reply to Stephen Webb', *The British Journal of Social Work,* 31(5): 552.

Smith, N.K. (1929) *Immanuel Kant's Critique of Pure Reason*. London: Macmillan.

Talbot-Smith, A. and Pollock, A.M. (2006) *The New NHS – A Guide*. London: Routledge.

Thomas, M. (2008) 'Cognitive behavioural dimensions of a therapeutic relationship', in S. Haugh and S. Paul (eds) *The Therapeutic Relationship – Perspectives and Theme*. Herefordshire: PCCS Books, pp. 92–103.

United Kingdom Public Health Association (2007) *Climates and Change – The Urgent Need to Connect Health and Sustainable Development*. London: UKPHA.

Van de Luitgaarden, G.M. (2009) 'Evidence-based practice in social work: lessons from judgement and decision making theory', *The British Journal of Social Work*, 39(2): 243–60.

Webb, S.A. (2001) 'Some considerations on the validity of evidence-based practice in social work', *The British Journal of Social Work*, 31(1): 57–79.

Woodroofe, K. (1961) *From Charity to Social Work*. London: Routledge and Kegan Paul.

2 Evidence-Based Practice within Values-Based Care

Pat Rose and Jan Gidman

There is no doubt that high-quality research has revolutionised the delivery of health care over the past century. For example, the introduction of aseptic techniques, antibiotics and immunisations has played a major part in the management of infection and infectious diseases whilst improved anaesthetics, imaging and microsurgery have changed the face of surgery. Thomas, Burt and Parkes (in Chapter 1) have described the emergence of evidence-based practice (EBP) within health and social care. This chapter explores in more depth the three elements of EBP, namely research, professional expertise and service user experience, and discusses how they are integrated to inform the concept of values-based care. It will be argued that the complexity of health and social care requires an integrated approach to EBP, which recognises and values research and the expertise of professionals and service users as evidence to inform professional practice.

Evidence-based Practice

In order to examine what is meant by EBP, it is useful to begin with the dictionary definition of evidence (Box 2.1). Here we see that evidence can arise from a number of sources. In terms of research, the first definition would apply; that is, available facts drawn from the data collected. However, evidence can also be information given by individuals such as would be used in a law court.

Box 2.1   Definitions of evidence

Evidence:

1. The available facts, circumstances, etc. Supporting or otherwise a belief, proposition, etc. Or indicating whether or not a thing is true or valid.
2. a. Information given personally or drawn from a document, etc. Tending to prove a fact or proposition.
   b. Statements or proofs admissible as testimony in a law court.
3. Clearness, obviousness.

Source: Concise Oxford Dictionary (1991)

In examining the meaning of evidence for health and social care provision, Lomas et al. (2005) undertook a systematic review in which they examined how the concept of 'evidence' was treated by those who produce the scientific evidence, those who formulate guidance such as guidelines, standards, benchmarks, targets, advisory reports and so on, and those who make decisions. They also reviewed articles that were about health-sector deliberative processes for combining different forms of evidence to produce guidance. Their analysis suggested that there are three views of what the 'evidence' in evidence-based practice is:

1. Evidence from medical effectiveness research which they call 'context-free scientific evidence'. This form of evidence relies on experimental research to establish universal truths which apply regardless of context.
2. Evidence associated with applied social sciences such as attitude studies, surveys and case studies which Lomas et al. (2005) describe as 'context-sensitive scientific research'. This relies on the realities of experts, stakeholders and others within a specific context.
3. Evidence described as colloquial evidence. This can be evidence about resources, expert and professional opinion, political judgement, values, habits and traditions, lobbyists and pressure groups, and the particular practicalities of not only a specific context but also a specific situation within that context. This is linked with the idea of evidence as the testimony of individuals.

Lomas et al. (2005) argue that these views of evidence are not incompatible and each has a role to play in EBP. However, combining them is a deliberative process which requires a high level of professional expertise.

This idea of the combining of scientific evidence with individual perceptions is at the heart of the original formulation of evidence-based medicine

(EBM), the precursor to EBP. In their seminal work on EBM, Sackett et al. (1997) define it as 'the conscientious, explicit and judicious use of current best evidence in making decisions about the care of individual service users' (p. 2). This is a familiar definition but in the same paragraph they suggest that the decision-making process in EBM involves 'integrating individual clinical expertise with best available external clinical evidence from systematic research'. Finally, and again in the same paragraph, they clarify further the meaning of clinical expertise as being acquired through experience, and involving the 'thoughtful identification and compassionate use of individual service users' predicaments, rights and preferences in making decisions about their care'. Clearly in this early exposition of the nature of EBM, the service user is central. This is reiterated when Sackett et al. (1997: 3) state that EBM 'requires a bottom-up approach that integrates the best external evidence with individual clinical expertise and service user choice'. Thus, a fundamental element of values-based care, respect for the wishes of the service user, was evident in EBP from the outset.

Evidence-based medicine originated at the McMaster University Medical School in Canada in the 1990s, and was a term used to describe a system of practice that appeared to lower the value of expert opinion and raise the value of rationalistic research. Gomm and Davies (2000) argue that, because randomised controlled trials (RCTs) control variables and therefore exclude confounding effects, they provide the closest we can get to certainty, and have become the gold standard for the evidence used in EBP. This has resulted in the seeming loss of the other elements that make up EBP, which, it is argued here, has led to a narrow perspective of evidence which does not recognise the valuable contribution of expertise from both professionals and service users. Welsh and Lyons (2001) support this view, reiterating that a reductionist approach to care cannot always encompass the wide-ranging and complex needs of service users, thus claiming that there is a case for basing practice on tacit knowledge, professional intuition and experience.

The Complexity of Health and Social Care

The complexity of health and social care provision encompasses the context of care provision, the multiple cultures of service users and their social settings, the individual care providers, and their profession's principles and values. Thus, as McCormack (2006) suggests, there is a need for a transformation of perspective, away from arguments about hierarchies of evidence towards integration of multiple forms of evidence. He argues that practice is 'messy, complex and enmeshed in ethical conflict' (p. 90).

To add to the argument, Macdonald (2000) comments that the term 'evidence-based' has been redefined, changing the nature of EBP as it was understood in health care, to allow for its increasing application to social care. In social care research, Pawson (2006) argues the case for meta-synthesis rather than meta-analysis. He is suggesting that in this context it is not reasonable to view an intervention as a potential cause of change as in health care, because a programme, unlike a drug, when implemented is dynamic; responsive to the service users, the social context, and the resources available. Thus, a meta-analysis of the outcomes of a social care programme will not be analysing the efficacy of a single entity but a range of interventions adapted to the context in which they were implemented. He goes on to propose a new model for meta-synthesis. This takes all the primary sources of evaluation of a social care programme and shows how its complex and interrelated elements can be used to initiate discussions about the future direction of the programme and inform social care policy making, particularly in respect of the effective use of resources.

Lomas et al. (2005), in their systematic review of how the concept of evidence was treated by various protagonists (detailed above), describe this type of discussion as a deliberative process which involves consultation with stakeholders and combines various types of evidence in order to reach an evidence-based decision. However, they found little evidence that the process is effective; partly because it is not neutral and may well influence the relative weight assigned to each of the three forms of evidence, thus influencing the extent to which any recommendations would be perceived as evidence-based by the parties involved. Nevertheless, they found that the characteristics of the process were likely to ensure any resulting guidance included consultation with all parties affected by the outcome, fair representation of scientists and stakeholders, and high-quality syntheses of all forms of evidence.

Traditional medical education focuses on competence (knowledge, skills and attitudes) but the current context of care requires more than this (Fraser and Greenhalgh, 2001). Thus, complexity theory is relevant to contemporary policy for education in the NHS to develop capability as well as competence (the ability to adapt to change, generate new knowledge and continuously improve performance). Sweeney and Kernick (2002) criticise the current reductionist paradigm in medicine, arguing that it does not incorporate human values, and they also advocate complexity theory as appropriate to medical education. These views could be applied to a varying degree in other health and social care education programmes (see Chapter 7).

Complexity theory recognises the interactions among the constituent elements in a system, and the addition of new elements or agents multiplies exponentially the number of potential connections and interactions within that system (Mason, 2008). Health and social care settings are constantly changing in terms of the agents within them; systems which include human agents have additional complexity in terms of their norms, values, language and narratives. The agents in health and social care organisations include a range of professionals, support staff, students, service users and carers.

It is argued that simplistic, linear models are not sufficient to explain the ways in which complex systems respond to the demands of the constantly changing, external environment. Neither the system nor its external environment are, or ever will be, constant. Uncertainty and paradox are inherent within them. These systems develop and change in order to survive, by means of networks and connections, self-organisation and emergence and their relationship with the external environment (Waldrop, 1992). This concept can readily be applied to health and social care organisations. As discussed in Chapter 1, there have been far-reaching changes within the systems in which health and social care are operating. Health and social care organisations may be considered as complex adaptive systems, in that they are unpredictable and non-linear, demonstrate emergent properties and rely on the relationships between their components.

Complexity theory may be an appropriate paradigm for the current policy drivers for health and social care, because it recognises the value, and indeed the necessity, of order and control for some aspects of care, whilst acknowledging and valuing the presence of uncertainty, rather than trying to exert control over other aspects of care. This provides a framework to address the potential tensions within professional practice, between the need for an evidence-based, competence-driven approach to ensure public safety and the empowerment of individuals, which recognises and values the knowledge gained from service user expertise.

Research as Evidence

In exploring how evidence informs policy, Davies and Nutley (2000) explicitly make the presumption that evidence means research, and they go on to summarise six reasons as to why rigorous research is necessary. These reasons are given below together with illustrative vignettes (2.1):

Vignette 2.1

1: Ineffective interventions abound

I feel dreadful, coughing, runny nose and headache. I went to my doctor for antibiotics but she would not give them to me. She told me I have a virus and antibiotics will not work.

2: Apparently logical therapies may be based on inadequate understanding of biological processes

My husband gets terrible depressions. Recently he had electric shock treatment and seemed much better so I looked up on the internet how it works. It says that it is not known why it works.

3: Some conditions spontaneously improve so there is a need to differentiate these from treatment-induced improvements

I have had a lot of back pain but I'm glad I didn't have the disc surgery I was offered because the pain has gone on its own.

4: Placebo effect when using expensive interventions needs to be identified

My sister has multiple-sclerosis but the doctor will not give her the latest drug. He says there is no evidence that people improve although it makes some feel better. I think feeling better is worth the price.

5: Small-scale studies can lead to erroneously accepting a therapy as efficacious, or erroneously rejecting a therapy as useless

I was in a project at the GP practice to see if service users lost weight if they attended a weekly advice session. Another group were just weighed weekly. Neither group lost much weight so now the advice sessions have been stopped.

6: Dangerous side effects of therapies need to be identified

There was a girl in my school who had missing arms because her mother had taken thalidomide during pregnancy.

Clearly, the research underpinning all these examples needs to be in the form of RCTs. Not all questions can be answered by experimentation and some accept that other research methodologies are necessary (Gomm and Davies, 2000). However, few acknowledge that there may be forms of evidence that are not research-based at all. The critical review of research as evidence for health and social care practice that follows, leads to consideration of the alternative perspectives offered by professional and service user expertise.

Social research as the underpinning evidence to support social care practice has been criticised as lacking the rigorous standards of health care practice. Macdonald (2000) argues that local research, such as surveys of service users' views, form a large part of the evidence for social care practices and that even nationally funded research with its 'preponderance of descriptive or exploratory studies, and evaluations using non-experimental designs' would not stand up to scrutiny in health care (Macdonald, 2000: 122). However, within this criticism, there is a failure to acknowledge that the problems encountered in social care are highly complex and do not arise from biological pathology that can be treated by technological or pharmacological interventions. Whilst the difficulties in applying the concept of EBP to social care include disagreement as to what constitutes evidence, and the antipathy towards RCTs, some of the strengths of research in social care which could be applied to health care are seen as:

- a wide range of validated approaches to service evaluation, particularly in service user opinion studies
- investment in research from the independent sector such as Barnardo's and the Joseph Rowntree Foundation
- overlaps with primary health care and therefore support from organisations such as the Cochrane Collaboration.

Thus, we see that the three aspects of EBP referred to earlier – research, professional expertise and service user expertise – complement each other to address the complexity of health and social care. Medicine's understanding of EBP based on RCTs and the meta-analysis of discreet diagnostic tools and interventions could be used by social care research to enhance the scientific rigour, where appropriate, and the meta-synthesis methods proposed as appropriate in social care could be used in health to answer the questions that do not lend themselves to experimentation and meta-analysis but nevertheless require rigorous study.

Those who argue that it is not appropriate to rely on research evidence alone, point to the way in which the context in which research is conducted is changing. For example, in response to growing concern regarding the difficulties in obtaining ethics approval for research, the British Medical Association (BMA) Medical Ethics Committee (2005: 3) presented a discussion paper focusing particularly on the issue of confidentiality and the use of service user data. In it, they argued that:

There are clearly benefits to society in conducting research for the future development of healthcare in the UK. Thus, society has an interest in promoting research and innovative treatment within an acceptable and workable framework. Such an acceptable framework, however, involves positively consulting service users whenever possible if identifiable data are used. This potentially raises problems for some research, particularly involving incapacitated or unconscious people. On the other hand impossibly high standards run the risk of pushing some research out of the UK.

In addition, they suggest that there are difficulties obtaining approval for retrospective research using data previously obtained for a different study, or data obtained from service users for therapeutic purposes, where the service users may be difficult or impossible to locate to give consent to the use of the data in research.

As more and more health and social care professions have moved their pre-qualification programmes into Higher Education Institutions (HEIs) and as promotion relies more and more heavily on post-qualification academic development, the pressure to publish has never been greater (Neuhauser et al., 2000). Whilst researchers may conduct their studies out of interest and for altruistic purposes, those working in HEIs aim to submit their research profiles for periodic national assessment (Higher Education Funding Council for England, 2009; RAE, 2008) in order to gain kudos and funding for their institution. It is argued that this pressure to publish, together with what some see as impossibly high ethical standards, has resulted in additional difficulties in assessing the quality of research findings beyond examining the rigour of such studies.

One of these difficulties is in assessing how up to date the research is. There is some evidence to suggest that studies with an outcome in favour of intervention will be published more quickly than studies with a negative outcome (Hopewell et al., 2007; Ioannidis, 1998; Stern and Simes, 1997). Duplicate publication is another problem in assessing the quality of research findings. The National Library of Medicine (NLM, 2008) of the United States defines a duplicate publication as 'an article that substantially duplicates another article without acknowledgement'. They go on to suggest that this 'may occur intentionally, to achieve wider dissemination of an article such as a policy statement, or inadvertently, through multiple submission of a manuscript to different journals'. However, Tramèr et al. (1997) argued that because of the pressure on academics to publish, there was a risk of deliberate covert duplicate publication of research findings. Whether accidental or deliberate, it does seem, however, that authors of systematic reviews are increasingly seeking and excluding duplicate data. Von Elm et al. (2004) found that of 141 systematic reviews related to anaesthesia and analgesia, 56 authors (40 per cent) had identified duplicate publication of data and had thus included it only once in their meta-analysis. However, on a more sombre note, in a recent study, Errami et al. (2008) examined the 607 articles annotated by the NLM up to July 2006 as duplicate publications and found that 42 per cent were true duplications. The others were updates, errata or comments which inadvertently duplicated the data. They went on to conduct a study of Medline citations using text similarity in titles and abstracts to compile a list of highly similar citations and reported that 1.35 per cent appeared to be duplicates. They concluded that, if this percentage was extrapolated to the entire database, 117,500 citations were likely to be covert duplicates. This indicates that duplicate publication, and the effect it has on meta-analysis, remains a problem.

Despite these issues, it is important to stress that research and the use of appropriate methods to implement it, remain vital components of the evidence required to underpin practice. It is, therefore, imperative not to dismiss the research element of EBP in favour of professional experience and service user choice, but rather to integrate all aspects of evidence.

One of the ways in which the consistent implementation of research evidence into practice has been promoted has been through the use of Integrated Care Pathways (ICPs). Middleton, Barnett and Reeves (2001: 1) define an ICP as 'a multidisciplinary outline of anticipated care, placed in an appropriate timeframe, to help a patient with a specific condition or set of symptoms move progressively through a clinical experience to positive outcomes'. They emphasise that the ICP must be 'patient-focused', providing appropriate care suitable for individual patients, and that it should provide a multi-disciplinary record of the input of each profession to the service user's care. NHS Scotland (2009) suggests ICPs are designed to reduce variation in practice and allow the same quality of care to be delivered to service users across multi-disciplinary and multi-agency teams and in different care settings. They plot the best sequence and timing of interventions by clinicians, nurses, other professionals and agencies for the best service user outcome and should be based on: evidence of good practice, patient experience, and professional experience and judgement. Interestingly, these are very similar to the three key features of EBP.

Though predominantly a feature of medicine, ICPs are also used by other health care professions. For example, McDonald (2005) describes how an ICP has facilitated collaboration between paediatricians and dentists to manage breathing difficulties in children. The Chartered Society of Physiotherapy (2002) recommend their development. In addition, there appears to be little doubt that ICPs are cost-effective in terms of shortening hospital stays, reducing costs and reducing prescribing errors (Cunningham et al., 2008; Olsson et al., 2009).

Whilst NHS Quality Improvement Scotland (2005) has placed an emphasis on the development of ICPs, particularly in the field of mental health care as part of its strategic work programme, the care pathways collection of the NHS for England and Wales (NHS Health Information Resources, 2009) has been switched off and an alternative, in the form of the Map of Medicine, replaces ICPs. These maps are web-based visual representations of evidence-based, service user care journeys covering 28 medical specialties and over 340 pathways. They differ from ICPs in that they do not provide documentation of care for individual service users, and thus do not provide a means for the audit of care outcomes. Nevertheless, they are evidence-based and support multi-professional collaboration.

As with any innovation, there are criticisms of ICPs. Some of the concerns are the same as those of any other form of guideline, for example they may limit professional freedom, they may lead to inflexibility and thus not meet individual service users' needs, they may need modification or supplements where service users have multiple needs, and they may even encourage litigation if they are not rigidly followed (Fisher and McMillan, 2004). A more serious issue is that some ICPs focus solely on medical treatment to the exclusion of all other aspects of service user well-being. For example, an ICP for the management of adults with methicillin-resistant staphylococcus aureus (MRSA) covers the identification of the site of infection, the level of cross-infection precautions needed, the range of topical and systemic medication needed and the duration of their use, and finally the process of confirmation that the service user is free of infection. What the ICP does not cover are factors such as the explanation of the condition, care and treatment of the service user, the support the service user will need when nursed in isolation and the education of visiting friends and family. Thus, this particular ICP appears to lack a multi-professional approach and any reference to the psychological needs of the service user.

Having explored the need for rigorous research to underpin health and social care practice, and some of the associated difficulties and dilemmas, this chapter will continue with a discussion of the role of professional expertise in EBP.

Professional Expertise

Returning to Sackett et al.'s (1997) definition of EBM, and the importance of professional judgement and clinical expertise, Rycroft-Malone (2006) argues that the regulation of health and social care practice through evidence-based guidelines erodes the very basis of professionalism by removing the opportunity for professional judgement in decision making regarding individual service users. The following vignette (2.2) illustrates the potential tension between guidelines, professional expertise and service user choice.

Vignette 2.2

I have been taking the same dose of thyroxin for over 15 years for an under-active thyroid gland. I have also been taking anti-depressants for two years which have allowed me to maintain an active retirement. As a retired nurse I am well aware of the importance of taking my medication and of reporting any changes in my condition to my GP.

I was annoyed when recently I was told that instead of my usual six-month supply of thyroxin, which has been dispensed since I was diagnosed many years ago, I can now have only three months supply at a time. This seems strange to me because the GP only checks my blood levels annually – so the prescription is not going to change is it?

I was also told that I could only have one month's supply of anti-depressant medication at a time. When I queried this with my GP she informed me, with a note of irritation in her voice, that this was due to 'guidelines'. I was told by a colleague that it is because some people with mental health problems do not take their medication regularly and it is way of monitoring this if they have to ask for a prescription every month. Also, she told me that it is not good to have a lot of drugs in a house where other people could get them.

I have been on prescribed medication for many years, I have always followed the prescription requirements and the evidence to support this is in my medical records. I live alone and the fact that I am well should be evidence enough that I have not let anyone else get hold of my drugs. My choice would be to have all the prescriptions at the same time, every three months. As I don't pay prescription charges it would be cheaper for the NHS for me to have bigger supplies and less stressful for me to collect all the prescriptions at once.

In this vignette, we see a deeply frustrated service user and a doctor who apparently feels that her practice is restricted by evidence-based guidelines. Rycroft-Malone (2006) goes so far as to argue that EBP is a means of controlling practitioners and that they need guidelines to tell them what to do because 'clinicians are either too busy or not skilled enough to find and interpret this knowledge for themselves' (p. 97). Whilst it is certainly true that health and social care professionals are very busy, and it is probably true that many of them do not have the skill to interpret the findings of often contradictory research studies, this does not mean that guidelines should be abandoned. Perhaps the doctor in this vignette is inexperienced, or over-zealous in her interpretation of the guidelines, viewing them as rules rather than guid-ance. Or perhaps she has had experiences that make her wary of trusting even the seemingly most conscientious of service users. If each encounter needs to be taken in the context of the individual service user and his or her circumstances, the same must also apply to each practitioner.

In a critique of EBM, Freeman and Sweeney (2001) undertook focus groups with a total of 19 GPs and, using content analysis of the discussions, identified issues relating to implementing evidence.

- Personal and professional experience. For example, in caring for service users with atrial fibrillation, one doctor had given anti-coagulation medication to a service user who subsequently died so she was put off using it. However, the grandfather of another doctor had died of the condition and was not taking an anti-coagulant so that doctor always prescribed it for his service users.
- The service user–doctor relationship, and the need to interpret the evidence in the context of the individual.
- A perceived tension between primary and secondary care. An example of this is the GP who, together with a service user, had taken the deci-sion to take the risk and not use medication to reduce blood pressure because the service user did not want the side-effects, however the hospital cardiologist was described as having written a 'stroppy' letter about this decision.
- Feelings evidence. For example, a diabetic service user had become increasingly anxious as the GP had continually changed his medication in order to achieve the optimum blood chemistry.
- Choice of words in consultations was described as influencing service users when they were given treatment options, for example a doctor said he would describe an anti-coagulant as rat poison if he wanted to put a service user off selecting it.
- Logistical problems. For example, a doctor described being reluctant to prescribe an anti-coagulant for an 88-year-old woman living in a very rural location because if she fell and bled, she would have dif-ficulty getting rapid treatment.

Perhaps in the light of our vignette (2.2), a further difficulty could be added, dealing with the service user who clearly wants to, and is able to, take more responsibility for his or her own care than the guidelines suggest. The potential challenges of service user expertise as evidence for practice will now be considered.

Naylor (1995) suggested that one of the grey areas in evidence-based practice is the problem of clinical opinion being contradictory to the evidence. He argued that new drugs and technology proliferate at an unprecedented pace, and sufficient research to allow for meta-analysis cannot keep up. This means that clinical opinion may be ahead of published research, or cost may have reduced for treatments considered prohibitive in guidelines based on available research. In addition, he suggests that clinicians hold differing philosophies regarding intervention in the absence of evidence. Some favour treatment whereas others favour non-intervention. If evidence is inconclusive regarding an intervention, some will recommend it anyway whereas others will not. Indeed, Rycroft-Malone (2001) argued that relatively few interventions in health care have been subject to rigorous research and proposed a framework for establishing consensus based on available research, but also expert opinion and service user experience to develop national guidelines for clinicians. Whilst this is a laudable ideal, it is difficult to see how this consensus could be achieved at national level.

We have already seen that the narrow definition of EBP, as a process of using research as the basis of practice, has broadened to mean the combining of scientific results with professional expertise. It could be argued that it is the process of reasoning that turns information from both research and professional experience into evidence as it is appraised and applied to the situation of individual service users. For this reason, Harbison (2006) argues that uncertainty is inherent within the concept of EBP. She continues that there are two ways of interpreting research-based evidence. One is by using intuition and involves rapid unconscious processing in order to come to a decision. The second approach is analytical where there is deliberate, conscious consideration of the literature. She also suggests that information is cumulative in that as further evidence emerges, such as the service user's response to an intervention, decisions made relating to that individual, and to the intervention itself, will change.

Thornton (2006: 2) gives definitions of clinical expertise and service user values which by substituting clinical with professional, and patient with service user, can be applied to the full range of health and social care professions (Box 2.2).

Box 2.2   Definitions of clinical expertise and
service user values

Thornton's (2006) definitions	Adapted definitions
Clinical expertise: the ability to use our clinical skills and past experience to rapidly identify each patient's unique health state and diagnosis, their individual risks and benefits of potential interventions, and their personal values and expectations.	**Professional expertise:** the ability to use professional skills and past experiences to rapidly identify each service user's unique health and/or social status, and identify his or her values and expectations, and establish risks and benefits to that person of potential intervention.
Patient values: the unique preferences, concerns and expectations each patient brings to a clinical encounter and which must be integrated into clinical decisions if they are to serve the patient.	**Service user values:** the unique preferences, concerns and expectations each service user brings to an encounter with a health or social care professional and which must be integrated into professional decision making in order to provide care.

Service user Expertise

As we have seen in Chapter 1, reforms to health and social care have been a major aspect of this government's policy since it came into power and published an extensive range of policies. These policies were developed in the context of widespread dissatisfaction with health and social care, to provide greater transparency and promote a more active notion of citizenship (Appleby and Rosete, 2003; Coulter, 2003; Health Service Ombudsman for England, 2003; Newman, 2001). A central theme of the government reforms is public involvement in all aspects of service design and delivery; and there are corresponding professional requirements to involve service users in education programmes.

Participation of service users in the design and delivery of all public services has been a key theme within the Labour government's approach to public sector reform (Chief Medical Officer, 2001). For example, one of the main threads of the numerous recommendations of the Kennedy enquiry into the deaths of children at Bristol Royal Infirmary (DH, 2000a) was that service users and carers must be fully involved in and at the heart of the NHS. The subsequent NHS plan (DH, 2000b) emphasised the need for service users to have more say in their treatment and more influence on the delivery of services: 'for the first time, service users will have a real say in the NHS. They will have new powers and more influence over the way the NHS works' (p. 12). This emphasis on service user involvement and choice has continued in recent publications, for example in the Darzi report (DH, 2008) which reinforces the need to value and meet the needs of each individual.

The government highlighted the threats to public trust in the NHS, particularly in relation to failures in communication and accountability and produced a policy to promote service user involvement at all levels (DH, 2003). It has also engaged in a range of listening and consultation exercises to explore public views and has increasingly used service user satisfaction surveys to influence care (Opinion Leader Research, 2006). This emphasises the highly political nature of the public services within the context of an ever-increasing gap between public expectations and actual provision (O'Neill, 2005). This emphasis on service user involvement assumes that service users have some kind of expert knowledge that is not available from other sources.

The expertise of service users is widely recognised (Beresford et al., 2005; Hasler, 2003). However, SCOPE (2005: 11), a voluntary organisation for people with disabilities, argues that 'the expertise of service users is possibly the most under utilised resource in social care'. They contend that current models of working with disabled people are limited, even tokenistic, with only a small group of individuals involved, and under-representation of black and ethnic minority groups, people with learning difficulties and those with mental health problems. Some ways in which this can be addressed are discussed in Chapter 6.

We have already identified the complexity of care provision in health and social care settings and have seen that, because of the way evidence-based practice has been defined, the context seems to have been neglected in favour of research evidence. Rycroft-Malone (2006) reminds us that the philosophical–normative orientation to evidence suggests that research evidence has inherent value on the basis of recognised measures of validity and reliability. However, the practical–operational orientation to evidence suggests that evidence is not static and is characterised by the decision-making context to which it relates. People are not passive recipients of evidence – they are stakeholders in the decision-making process.

Complexity theory has been applied to knowledge acquisition in general medical practice by Sweeney (2006). He explains that medicine mirrors the two fundamental characteristics of science: linearity and reductionism, and that this has traditionally relied on the rationalist–positivist ontology. He contends that currently, in medicine, statistical and clinical significance are used to assess the value of knowledge and he argues for the recognition of a third level of significance, that is, personal significance: 'At stake in the definition of that third level – personal significance – is the centrality of subjectivity and interaction, and of emergence in the clinical encounter. We are forced to consider that this represents a different "way of knowing"' (Sweeney, 2006: 44). Furthermore, Griffiths (2002) advises that complexity theory provides a framework to understand and value the knowledge gained from a specific service user, in a specific context. It supports the value of service users' stories which are said to promote an understanding of service users' perspectives.

Complex medical consultations, where traditional biomedical knowledge is insufficient, are discussed by Fraser and Greenhalgh (2001) who suggest that learning occurs in the zone of complexity. They suggest that, within this zone of complexity, 'relationships between items of knowledge are not predictable or linear but neither are they frankly chaotic. Learning which builds capability takes place when individuals engage with uncertain and unfamiliar contexts in a meaningful way' (Fraser and Greenhalgh, 2001: 800). Thus, service user involvement is not merely a panacea to a more enquiring public, to make them feel involved. Service user experience is an essential part of the evidence to support health and social care interventions.

A recent study by one of this chapter's authors (Gidman, 2009) identified that student nurses, midwives and social workers used alternative forms of knowledge, particularly service user and client stories, to learn in practice settings. All of the respondents in the study accessed a range of individual service users during their practice placements, and used this knowledge to influence their practice. All the respondents described their learning from critical incidents, service users' stories, interactions with service users and observing role models. From this, they developed their own philosophies of professional ideals and professional roles, including the nature of effective relationships and understanding service users' perspectives. The students valued humanistic, authentic relationships between professionals and service users and recognised the inappropriate use of professional power. This is consistent with the health and social care policies discussed above (and in Chapter 6), which promote the active involvement of service users in all aspects of health and social care planning, delivery and evaluation. The data suggest that students, in this study, listened to and valued service users' perspectives of their situations and provided opportunities for them to tell their stories and to maintain responsibility for their own health and illness.

An example of the data from this study (Vignette 2.3) illustrates how a social work student learned from listening to the story of a woman with a long history of mental health problems.

> ## Vignette 2.3
>
> I think, first of all I try to get to know a person, so I'm not going in with any, sort of, preconceived thoughts or ideas. Erm, she was quite mentally ill, and you know, just her look – you could see that she was mentally ill and I didn't want that to get in the way. So, I do try very hard to let the person come out if you like, and so it was spending the first few times just listening, just basically listening and for me to try to get an understanding of her perspective on things. Which she did very well, she had tremendous insight into her own experiences, into the way other people experience her and either understand her or not. You know – the fear that people have – she talked about all that really openly. I would imagine it's quite easy for a person who becomes mentally ill – to try and take over their thoughts and actions for them – because you feel that they are not in a position to be able to do it rationally … and while there might be periods when she might not be rational, she still knows what's going on, and she'll remember it once she comes out of that stage. She was on about, when she gets put in hospital, she is fearful of bathing or washing her hair … she'll have a strip wash in the morning but she never wants to wash her hair and she's got very long hair, and when she goes into hospital … 'nobody appreciates how frightened I am … that water, around me, it really makes me frightened'. She really taught me loads … her understanding, her level of understanding.

Stories have been advocated as strategies both to empower service users, and as an alternative form of knowledge. Birth stories, for example, are recognised in midwifery education as a valuable tool to help women understand their experiences of childbirth, and more recently to promote learning for students (Farley and Widmann, 2001). In his influential work *The Wounded Storyteller*, Frank (1997) proposes that storytelling can help the service user move from a passive to an active role in his or her illness. He contends that illness greatly affects the person's '… sense of where she is in life and where she may be going. Stories are a way of redrawing maps and finding new destinations' (Frank, 1997: 53). Service users' stories are said to be valuable, often unrecognised, tools to tap into students' imaginations, form meaningful connections, promote learning and enhance reflection (Greenhalgh and Collard, 2003). Although there are a range of different meanings in the education context, it is argued that stories can be 'a vehicle to facilitate learning rather than to impart knowledge' (Moon and Fowler, 2008: 232).

Hallenbeck (2003) suggests that professionals and service users have different types of stories. The stories from professionals value objective and rational perspectives and those of service users and their families value subjective and emotional perspectives. Hallenbeck (2003) illustrates this by referring to his own experiences with service users in the context of palliative care, highlighting the different perspectives that medical staff and service users and their families have of the same situation. Cox (2001) proposes that stories are a valuable aspect of medical education. He suggests that service user stories can promote the development of professional expertise and provide a framework to link the objective and subjective knowledge inherent in complex case management. These stories, then, form a crucial element of evidence and together with evidence from research in all its forms, and from professional expertise, move us beyond the current narrow view of evidence-based practice to one that celebrates the complexity of the human experience of both professionals and service users in health and social care contexts.

Conclusion

Ten years ago, Batstone and Edwards (1998) argued that there are too many critics of EBP to sideline them as laggards in the process of introducing EBP. Over the years, increasing attention has been given to their opinions. This chapter has discussed a range of those opinions. The value of RCTs, as evidence to underpin medical practice, has been acknowledged, but it has been argued that other forms of research, for example those used widely in social studies, also provide valuable evidence for professional practice. The chapter has considered potential issues in relation to research as evidence and suggested that professional and service user expertise should also be recognised and used to inform practice. This integrated approach to evidence is required to address the complexity of health and social care practice. This supports Sackett et al.'s (1997: 3) original view, referred to earlier in this chapter, that EBP 'requires a bottom-up approach that integrates the best external evidence with individual clinical expertise and service user choice'. However, the potential tensions between these three forms of evidence and the difficulties associated with developing national guidelines using this integrated approach are acknowledged. In the following chapters, the discussion will further explore how values-based care aims to retain the positive aspects of EBP but incorporate the missing elements.

References

Appleby, J. and Rosete, A. (2003) 'The NHS: keeping up with public expectations?', in A. Park, J. Curice, K. Thomson, L. Jarvis and C. Bromley (eds) *British Social Attitudes: The 20th Report – Continuity and Change over Two Decades*, p. 3. London: Sage.

Batstone, G. and Edwards, M. (1998) 'Coping with uncertainty in evidence-based practice', *Journal of Clinical Effectiveness*, 3(1): 1.

Beresford, P., Shamash, M., Forrest, V. and Turner, M. (2005) *Developing Social Care: Service Users' Vision for Adult Support*. London: Social Care Institute for Excellence.

BMA Medical Ethics Committee (2005) *Confidentiality as Part of a Bigger Picture – A Discussion Paper from the BMA*, Available at: www.bma.org.uk/images/confidentiality_tcm41-20480.pdf [accessed 1 December 2009]

Chartered Society of Physiotherapy (2002) *Integrated Care Pathways*. London: Chartered Society of Physiotherapy.

Chief Medical Officer (2001) *The Expert Service User: A New Approach to Chronic Disease Management for the 21st Century*. London: Department of Health.

Concise Oxford Dictionary (1991) Oxford: Oxford University Press.

Coulter, A. (2003) *The Autonomous Service User: Ending Paternalism in Medical Care*. London: The Stationery Office.

Cox, K. (2001) 'Stories as case knowledge', *Medical Education*, 35: 862–6.

Cunningham, S., Logan, C., Lockerbie, L., Dunn, M., McMurray, A. and Prescott, R. (2008) 'Effect of an integrated care pathway on acute asthma/wheeze in children attending hospital: cluster randomized trial', *The Journal of Pediatrics*, 152(3): 315–20.

Davies, H. and Nutley, S. (2000) 'Healthcare: evidence to the fore', in H. Davies, S. Nutley and P. Smith (eds) *What Works? Evidence-based Policy and Practice in Public Services*. Bristol: The Policy Press, pp. 43–68.

Department of Health (DH) (2000a) Kennedy Report into Deaths Following Paediatric Cardiac Surgery at Bristol Royal Infirmary. Bristol Royal Infirmary Inquiry, UK. London: Department of Health.

Department of Health (DH) (2000b) *The NHS Plan: A Plan for Investment, A Plan for Reform*. London: Department of Health.

Department of Health (DH) (2003) *Service User and Public Involvement in the New NHS*. London: Department of Health.

Department of Health (DH) (2008) *High Quality Care for All. NHS Next Stage Review: Final Report*. London: Department of Health.

Errami, M., Hicks, J.M., Fisher, W., Trusty, D., Wren, J.D., Long, T.C., Garner, H.R. (2008) 'Déjà vu – a study of duplicate citations in Medline', *Bioinformatics*, 24(2): 243–9.

Farley, C. and Widmann, S. (2001) 'The value of birth stories', *International Journal of Childbirth Education*, 16(3): 22–6.

Fisher, A. and McMillan, R. (2004) *Integrated Care Pathways for Day Surgery Patients*. Norwich: British Association of Day Surgery.

Frank, A.W. (1997) *The Wounded Storyteller: Body Illness and Ethics*. Chicago, IL: University of Chicago Press.

Fraser, S.W. and Greenhalgh, T. (2001) 'Coping with complexity: educating for capability', *British Medical Journal*, 323: 799–802.

Freeman, A.C. and Sweeney, K. (2001) 'Why General Practitioners do not implement evidence: qualitative study', *British Medical Journal*, 323: 1–5.

Gidman, J. (2009) *A Phenomenological Investigation of Nursing, Midwifery and Social Work Students' Perceptions of Learning from Patients and Service Users in Practice Settings*. PhD thesis, University of Liverpool.

Gomm, R. and Davies, C. (2000) *Using Evidence in Health and Social Care*. London: Sage.

Greenhalgh, T. and Collard, A. (2003) *Narrative Based Health Care: Sharing Stories – A Multi-Professional Workbook*. Oxford: Blackwell BMJ Publishing.

Griffiths, F. (2002) 'Conclusion', in K. Sweeney and F. Griffiths (eds) *Complexity and Healthcare: An Introduction*. Oxford: Radcliffe.

Hallenbeck, J. (2003) *Palliative Care Perspectives*. New York: Oxford University Press.

Harbison, J. (2006) 'Clinical judgement in the interpretation of evidence: a Baysian approach', *Journal of Clinical Nursing*, 15: 1489–97.

Hasler, F. (2003) *Users at the Heart: User Participation in the Governance and Operations of Social Care Regulatory Bodies*. London: Social Care Institute for Excellence.

Health Service Ombudsman for England (2003) *Annual Report HC700*. London: Parliamentary and Health Service Ombudsman.

Higher Education Funding Council for England (2009) *Research Excellence Framework*. Available at: www.hefce.ac.uk/research/ref/ [accessed 16 November 2009]

Hopewell, S., Clarke, M.J., Stewart, L. and Tierney, J. (2007) 'Time to publication for results of clinical trials', *Cochrane Database of Systematic Reviews 2007*, Issue 2. Art. No. MR000011. DOI: 10.1002/14651858. MR000011.pub2

Ioannidis J. (1998) 'Effect of the statistical significance of results on the time to completion and publication of randomised efficacy trials', *Journal of the American Medical Association*, 279: 281–6.

Lomas, J., Culyer, T., McCutcheon, C., McAuley, L. and Law, S. (2005) *Conceptualizing and Combining Evidence for Health System Guidance*. Ontario: Canadian Health Services Research Foundation.

McCormack, B. (2006) 'Evidence-based practice and the potential for transformation', *Journal of Research in Nursing*, 11(2): 89–94.

Macdonald, G. (2000) 'Social care: rhetoric and reality', in H. Davies, S. Nutley and P. Smith (eds) *What Works? Evidence-based Policy and Practice in Public Services*. Bristol: The Policy Press, pp. 117–40.

McDonald, J.P. (2005) 'The role of the dental surgeon in an integrated care pathway for the treatment of breathing difficulties', *British Dental Journal*, 19(8): 449.

Mason, M. (2008) 'What is complexity theory and what are its implications for educational change?', *Educational Philosophy and Theory*, 40(1): 35–49.

Middleton, S., Barnett, J. and Reeves, D. (2001) *What is an Integrated Care Pathway?* Newmarket: Hayward Medical Communications.

Moon, J. and Fowler, J. (2008) 'There is a story to be told: a framework for the conception for story in higher education and professional development', *Nurse Education Today*, 28: 232–9.

National Library of Medicine (NLM) (2008) *Errata, Retractions, Partial Retractions, Corrected and Republished Articles, Duplicate Publications, Comments (including Author Replies), Updates, Service User Summaries, and Republished (Reprinted) Articles Policy for MEDLINE®*. Factsheet. Available at: www.nlm.nih.gov/pubs/factsheets/errata.html#duplicate [accessed 1 December 2009]

Naylor, C.D. (1995) 'Grey zones of clinical practice: some limits to evidence-based medicine', *The Lancet*, 345(8953): 840–2.

Neuhauser, D., McEachern, E., Zazanski, S., Flocke, S. and Williams, R.L. (2000) 'Continuous quality improvement and the process of writing for academic publication', *Quality Management in Health Care*, 8(3): 65–73.

Newman, J. (2001) *Modernising Governance: New Labour, Policy and Society*. London: Sage.

NHS Health Information Resources (2009) *Protocols and Care Pathways (De-commissioned)*. London: NHS Health Information Resources. Available at: www.library.nhs.uk/pathways. [accessed 16th November 2009]

NHS Quality Improvement Scotland (2005) *Improving the Quality of Mental Health Services in Scotland*. Edinburgh: NHS Quality Improvement Scotland.

NHS Scotland (2009) *What are Integrated Care Pathways?* Edinburgh: NHS Scotland: Available at www.clinicalgovernance.scot.nhs.uk/section2/pathways.asp [accessed 16 November 2009]

Olsson, L., Hansson, E., Ekman, I. and Karlsson, J. (2009) 'A cost-effectiveness study of a patient-centred integrated care pathway', *Journal of Advanced Nursing*, 65(8): 1626–35.

O'Neill, F. (2005) 'Strategic direction of service user involvement in education', in T. Warne and S. McAndrew (eds), *Using Service User Experience in Nurse Education*. Basingstoke: Palgrave MacMillan, pp. 43–61.

Opinion Leader Research (2006) *Your Health, Your Care, Your Say: A Research Report*. London: Department of Health.

Pawson, R. (2006) *Evidence-based Policy: A Realist Perspective*. London: Sage.

Research Assessment Exercise (RAE) (2008) Available at: www.rae.ac.uk/ [accessed 1st December 2009]

Rycroft-Malone, J. (2001) 'Formal consensus: the development of a national clinical guideline', *Quality in Health Care*, 10(4): 202–3.

Rycroft-Malone, J. (2006) 'The politics of the evidence-based practice movements', *Journal of Research in Nursing*, 11(2): 95–108.

Sackett, D., Richardson, W., Rosenberg, W. and Hynes, R.B. (1997) *Evidence-based Medicine*. Edinburgh: Churchill Livingstone.

SCOPE (2005) *Scope's Response to the Green Paper, Independence, Well-being and Choice*. Available at: www.scope.org.uk/downloads/issues/ascgp_response.doc [accessed 1 December 2009]

Stern, J.M. and Simes, R.J. (1997) 'Publication bias: evidence of delayed publication in a cohort study of clinical research projects', *British Medical Journal*, 315(7109): 640–5.

Sweeney, K. (2006) *Complexity in Primary Care*. Oxford: Radcliffe.

Sweeney, K. and Kernick, D. (2002) 'Clinical evaluation: constructing a new model for post-normal medicine', *Journal of Evaluation in Clinical Practice*, 8: 131–8.

Thornton, T. (2006) 'Tacit knowledge as the unifying factor in evidence based medicine and clinical judgement', *Philosophy, Ethics and Humanities in Medicine*, 1(2). Available at: www.peh-med.com/content/1/1/2 [accessed 1 December 2009]

Tramèr, M.R., Raynolds, D.J.M., Moore, R.A. and McQuay, H.J. (1997) 'Impact of covert duplicate publication on meta-analysis: a case study', *British Medical Journal*, 315(7109): 635–40.

Von Elm, E., Poglia, G., Walder, B. and Tramèr, M.R. (2004) 'Different patterns of duplicate publication: an analysis of articles used in systematic reviews', *Journal of the American Medical Association*, 291(8): 974–80.

Waldrop, M. (1992) *Complexity: The Emerging Science at the Edge of Order and Chaos*. New York: Simon and Schuster.

Welsh, I. and Lyons, C.M. (2001) 'Evidence-based care and the case for intuition and tacit knowledge in clinical assessment and decision making in mental health nursing practice: an empirical contribution to the debate', *Journal of Psychiatric and Mental Health Nursing*, 8: 299–305.

3 Caring: Values and Evidence

Pat Rose and Sue Phillips

'Care is not an aspect of treatment that may or may not enhance clinical outcomes; care is the reason for giving treatment to another person' (Olsen, 2000: 470), thus caring should be the fundamental value espoused by all health and social care professionals. In 2005, of the approximate 1.3 million people working in the NHS, 679,157 were professionally qualified clinical staff and a further 376,219 were support workers to clinical staff (The Information Centre, 2006). Add to this the one million plus social care workforce (DH, 2009a) and we have a workforce of over 2.3 million paid workers providing health and social care to the British population. In addition, there is an unknown number of carers, defined by the Social Care Institute for Excellence (SCIE, 2007: 4) as 'people who provide unpaid care to a relative, friend or neighbour who is in need of support because of mental or physical illness, old age or disability' who supplement the professional care services. In this chapter, the focus is on caring as applied to the role of health and social care professionals who provide a service either directly to service users, or to their carers; this was a topic high on the government agenda in the late 2000s (Age Concern, 2005; Standing Commission on Carers, 2009). However, much of the discussion applies to caring in any context.

The nature of caring has exercised the minds of philosophers and health and social care professionals alike. In nursing in particular, it has been a recurrent theme, some even claiming 'caring to be synonymous with nursing' (Wilkin and Slevin, 2004: 50). As recently as 2008, Corbin asked the question: 'Is caring a lost art in nursing?' (p. 163). This generated a lengthy discussion through the pages of the journal which Rolfe (2009) eventually commented uses the term 'caring' in four distinct ways, namely:

- a generic term for nursing practice, i.e. nursing care
- a term for a particular aspect of practice such as palliative care or technical medical care
- a very specific term for the ineffable art of 'caring about' that sometimes accompanies the more technical 'caring for'
- the 'complete package' of caring about *and* caring for.

Rolfe went on to suggest that there is a need to continue to use the term caring, recognising that in the absence of anything better or more precise, we are keeping alive the several different and contradictory meanings that it simultaneously signifies, and the necessity to continue talking about it whilst recognising that we might not all be discussing the same concept.

Barker (2000) describes the idea of care as a 'crafted object', having a human aesthetic quality, but also depending on the exercise of a skill or technique which equates it to a science. However, Barker points out that care, as a crafted object, is dependent on the context in which it takes place and it gains its meaning through the interaction of those being cared for and those undertaking the caring. Engster (2007) applied this view more specifically to the caring professions. He described the two ways of caring in relation to, first, virtue-based definitions which focus on the internal motivations and intentions of the care-givers and, secondly, practice-based definitions which emphasise external actions and their consequences. Engster argues that neither approach on its own represents true care. For example, one can bath a person either in a way that demonstrates care for the person, or demonstrates total disinterest in the person, or one can fully intend to help someone bath, but not actually do it. This chapter thus begins by exploring caring as a science and how this links with evidence-based practice. It will then review some of the accounts of philosophers and others regarding the nature of caring. The art of caring is then examined in more detail in relation to the theory of art and the way it relates to human values.

The study of caring has been undertaken within both the rationalistic and naturalistic paradigms. Kyle (1995) examined the findings of a range of studies from both paradigms and found that although both have limitations, both show similar findings. The literature she reviewed showed that health and social care professionals tended to value the affective elements of caring, driven by emotions, such as providing comfort through listening. However, the service users tended to value the behavioural elements requiring knowledge and skill rooted in research evidence, such as knowing how to give injections and when to call a doctor. Various reasons for this are given, for example behavioural skills involve meeting basic physiological needs whilst the affective domain relates to higher needs, or that service users assume the affective elements are natural and therefore not specifically a role of the professional. Whatever the reasons, it is important to note that service users perceive the caring professional as competent, skilled and knowledgeable.

Distinctions are made between caring *for* someone caring *about* someone and caring *with* someone (Barker, 2000). Dunlop (1986) suggests that a science *for* caring involves applying the findings of science to achieve the ends determined by caring, for example by researching areas of knowledge from public health, epidemiology, physiology, biology, psychology and social psychology. A science *of* caring implies that caring can be operationalised in some way as a set of behaviours which can be observed, counted or measured. Curative factors and caring constructs, Dunlop argues, are not context free, for example comfort, compassion and concern are highly dependent on the context. Dunlop suggests that the only way to elucidate 'caring' is to take a hermeneutic form, citing Benner's (1984) work on nursing as an example. What this can do is describe the sorts of things that good carers do; and how they work out their caring in practice.

Sack (2006) suggests that if caring is the critical outcome of our health and social care system, it should be subject to scientific study, like other outcomes. However, the question is whether caring can be dissected into crucial elements that may be more amenable to study. Sack proposes that three of these elements may include 'commitment', 'connections' and 'compassion'. He looks at these three to see if there may be a scientific approach to their study, however he does not state the types of study that may be applied to attempt to quantify these elements. Dunlop (1986) argues that caring cannot be subjected to traditional scientific enquiry without distorting it past recognition, as caring is not seen to reside in a set of practices, but in a thinking–feeling mode of being which gives rise to activity, including the choice of refraining from activity.

Sturgeon (2008) considers the implications of over-emphasising the role of interpersonal relationships and emotional engagement in caring, and argues that there should be a balance between interpersonal and technical skills. The importance of scientific knowledge is substantiated by, for example, the accounts of successful resuscitation of near-drowned children. Knowledgeable practitioners argue to continue resuscitation on the basis of scientific knowledge of the effect of hypothermia in this situation, not on the emotional grounds of the overwhelming tragedy of a lost child. However, Appleton and Cowley (2008) found that health visitors, when undertaking health needs assessment, drew on more than scientific knowledge of child health and development and post-natal depression, as illustrated in Vignette 3.1.

Vignette 3.1

After my second baby was born, she wouldn't settle. Feeding seemed to take forever and she never seemed to be satisfied and cried all the time. My toddler, Mike, was playing up and I was at the end of my tether with lack of sleep and so on. No one seemed to understand. My health visitor, Trisha, came and gave me a questionnaire to fill in about post-natal depression. I knew what the right answers should be, so I filled it in accordingly, as I didn't think I was depressed, it was just the children being difficult. However, Trisha sat and talked with me; she seemed to have plenty of time, which surprised me. I gradually found myself opening up to her about how difficult I was finding things and how I wasn't coping with the baby and Mike. She showed me on their charts that both Mike and the baby were developing well. She was very calm, and helped me to understand what was going on, and that I might actually have post-natal depression. This was a turning point for me, and helped get things in perspective. I got help from my doctor, my family supported me. Trisha knew I was depressed but I would not admit it. It was only because she really cared that I finally let her in.

Evidence for practice may be applied on the basis of considerations of utility (Mulhall cited by Seymour et al., 2003). However, Quinney et al., (1997) question the advice to withdraw from the NHS some clinical procedures which have been shown to have no evidence base or to be of doubtful utility or outcome. It is argued that the rational, technical goal, with its focus on measurable activity and tasks, is being pursued at the expense of more holistic, supportive and softer aspects of health and social care which may not be so tangible and easily quantifiable, but are more associated with the humanistic idea of caring. This is discussed in more detail in Chapter 2 where the concept and efficacy of evidence-based practice is analysed.

Little (2002: 319) describes humanistic medicine as 'a term compounded, for therapeutic purposes, with the good intent of reminding clinicians of their need to be compassionate and empathic'. McConnell (cited by Musk, 2004) suggests that the competing demands of choosing between time for high-technology procedures and time for caring may mean the need for a balancing act, or compromise between procedures and caring. However, this seems to suggest that technological tasks and caring are mutually exclusive. Musk (2004) argues that health and social care professionals can retain a caring humanistic approach, independent of technological competence. However, Ray (cited by Musk, 2004) claims that caring is technical competence and Locsin (cited by Musk, 2004) concludes that technological incompetence is tantamount to not caring. Hawthorne and Yurkovich (1995) believe that the perceived decreased level of caring in the professions is due to an over-emphasis on science and technology. They suggest the need for a spiritual dimension to caring to engage with others on an individual basis. Arthur, et al., (2001) assert that the more technology influences the relationship between service users and health and social care professionals, the more the professionals need to demonstrate caring attributes, such as communication and involving the service user in decision making. In fact, their comparative study found that nurses working in a highly technological environment displayed more of these caring attributes than nurses working in low technology environments. Interestingly, advocacy as a caring attribute scored higher in the low technology environments. Vignette 3.2 illustrates the way a service user felt about a nurse who actually ignored evidence related to infection control to provide immediate care. Whilst the profession would not advocate the removal of sutures in this way, for the service user it was the approach of the nurse that mattered more.

Vignette 3.2

I had one long stitch in my tummy, with a little blue bead each end. I was very nervous about it being taken out so I screwed up my eyes and said 'Do it now'. The nurse said it might feel a bit odd or tingly but it shouldn't hurt. Then she asked me if I wanted her to do it bit by bit, or in one go. I asked her to do it in one go, and I couldn't resist looking – I think so I could stop her if it hurt. She then opened a little packet with a cutter in it. She took one of the beads and cut just below it, then she took the other bead and gently but deftly pulled the stitch out and I didn't feel a thing. It was only afterwards that I realised she had not worn gloves and had used her fairly long fingernails to hold the beads. But that didn't matter, she did the things that mattered, told me what would happen and asked me what I wanted. I think if she had gone off to get equipment like gloves and forceps that would have scared me more. She was one of the really good nurses on the ward.

Both Malterud (2001) and Nay (2003) point out that evidence-based practice, as defined by purists, speaks largely of scientific evidence being the result of randomised controlled trials, with surveys, cohort studies and case studies coming in as second best. For them, qualitative studies do not count as evidence. However, these authors argue that the caring professions require more than just the results of controlled experiments in the practice of their disciplines, because real-life scenarios are not controlled situations; there are a multitude of individual variances which need interpretation by the practitioner. As Brilowski and Wendler (2005) note, caring may be dependent on the circumstances, the environment and the people involved: an attribute of caring that they describe as 'variability'. This suggests that there cannot be a single statement that accurately defines caring. However, there have been a number of attempts by philosophers, nurses and others to define it, often using a reductionist approach in which caring is defined through describing a series of characteristics that can be ascribed to it (Box 3.1).

Box 3.1   Defining attributes of caring

Mayeroff (1971)	Roach (1987)	Swanson (1991)	Brilowski and Wendler (2005)	Morse et al. (1990)	Wolf et al. (1994)
Knowing	Compassion	Knowing	Relationship	Human	Respectful
Alternating rhythms	Competence	Being with	Action	trait	deference
Patience	Confidence	Doing for	Attitude	Moral	to others
Honesty	Conscience	Enabling	Acceptance	imperative	Assurance
Trust	Commitment	Maintaining belief	Variability	Affect	of human
Humility				Interpersonal	presence
Hope				relationship	Positive
Courage				Therapeutic	connectedness
				intervention	Professional knowledge
					Attentiveness to other's experience
					and skill

Caring is a particular emotional and behavioural response that draws on technical and interpersonal knowledge and skills. Roach (1987) identifies 'compassion', 'conscience' and 'commitment' as the emotional element, whilst 'competence' and 'confidence' relate to the behavioural response. In Swanson's (1991) five categories of caring, 'doing for' is clearly a behavioural response and 'being with' is the emotional response. The behavioural response alone – engaging with and doing things for people in a competent and knowledgeable way – is not always done in a caring way. It is the integration of the emotional element within the behaviour that defines an action as caring.

Malterud (2001) argues that even taken-for-granted medical tasks, such as the reading of mammographic images, are not completely scientifically proven; they are subject to individual interpretation. It is the 'tacit knowledge' of an experienced practitioner that is needed to supplement the scientific results when undertaking clinical decision making. For example, Nay (2003: 342) states: 'if EBP is to improve care outcomes for older people, it must also be informed by care context, service user preferences, and clinical judgement based on individualized assessments and care plans'. Through asking service users in London about their experiences, Age Concern (2005) claimed that professional care and care services in London were failing elderly people. In this context, 'care services' refer to professional carers rather than lay carers. The ways in which the services were deemed to be failing were:

- restricted access to care and support
- limited choice and control over care services, for example 'with home care, older people have little say about what is to be done, when and by whom' (p. 3)
- being put at risk from untrained and unqualified staff. It was claimed that 'Although more care staff are gaining qualifications that demonstrate their competence, the majority are still unqualified' and that 'many care service managers and commissioners lack the necessary skills and knowledge for their roles' (p. 3)
- hardship caused by inadequate funding and controversy about who pays for long-term care.

However, as in most situations, the care providers themselves may have a different perspective leading to a lack of congruence between the perceptions of the carer, who has to consider all those needing care, and the service user who only knows his or her own needs. This is illustrated in Vignette 3.3.

Vignette 3.3

This week Janet's on holiday so they sent another carer, Rene. She seems nice enough, but she's rather bossy. I think she must have been in a hurry. She says things like, 'Come on, Joan, let's get you into the bath now, and then you can have your lunch'. I explained my usual routine, that if I'm in a lot of pain, it's better to let the pills

(continued)

(Continued)

work before moving me too much. Rene says it will suit her better, as she has other people to go to. Janet always asks before moving me, she seems to have more time. I'll be so glad when she's back on Monday.

In this case, Rene may genuinely have much less time than Janet as she has to do Janet's work as well as her own. Also, doing things differently does not necessarily mean a lack of care. Rene's view of caring may be more related to efficiency for the whole case load. She may also have felt that the service user was procrastinating over her bath in order to keep the carer there longer, rather than actually being in pain. However, the self-aware professional would reflect on the encounter afterwards and try to work out a compromise between her perception, what the service user asked for, and the needs of other service users. Kenny (1997) suggests that clinical practice is both science and art, and that clinical judgement, the creative element of practice, is poorly understood and often based on idiosyncratic opinion. Simply breaking caring down into a series of defining attributes does little to help. What is needed is an understanding of the relationship between the application of science and the art of caring.

In examining what caring actually is, Mayeroff (1971) lists eight major ingredients (Box 3.1). Interestingly, his first ingredient is 'knowing'. He says that 'in order to care I must understand the other's needs and must be able to respond properly' (p. 19). For evidence-based professions, the importance of knowledge in health and social care is paramount. Roach (1987) equates competence with an appropriate level of knowledge and skill. Swanson (1991) expands on this to suggest that a caring professional will avoid assumptions and seek to understand the meaning of a situation in the life of the service user, something the doctor caring for Mary did not achieve (Vignette 3.4).

Vignette 3.4

My name is Mary. I was recovering from abdominal surgery to treat endometriosis, a painful and debilitating condition. My intravenous drip had stopped working, the nurse had removed it and a doctor had come to put a new one in. The doctor was having difficulty finding a vein because I am fat. At one point he said

(Continued)

(Continued)

'once you get home you will need to do more exercise then you'll have veins like Arnold Schwarzenegger'. I burst into tears and he talked to me as though I was crying because of the discomfort of the needle. I tried to explain, through my tears, that I was not squeamish nor worried by needles. I was crying because I had got fat, because I had become more immobile and very tired due to pain. My beloved garden was a mess and my home uncared for. I felt as though he was blaming me for him not being able to find a vein.

To fully understand the meaning of the situation for the service user, the professional must undertake a thorough assessment. This presupposes a detailed knowledge of the range of normal human experience and an ability to identify any health-related deviations. The focus of assessment is to understand the needs of others, but responding to those needs requires knowledge of interventions and how to implement them. Thus, the caring professional will be an educated person who keeps up to date with changes and developments in practice. The problem with Mary's story is that the doctor may not have known that she perceived him as uncaring. He was probably becoming a little stressed by the difficulty he was experiencing in putting the needle in and tried to relieve the tension through humour. He may never have met Mary before and almost certainly had not read her notes in detail. In this case, the attempt at caring failed. For another service user, however, exactly the same technique may have proved successful. In terms of art, perhaps this equates with personal taste, and the fact that not everyone will be moved by the same work of art. For example, Yves Klein's painting of a blue rectangle, entitled 'Blue' (DLA Piper, 2008), may leave some people cold whilst others are strongly moved by it.

'Alternating rhythms' is Mayeroff's (1971) second major ingredient of caring. He suggests that the carer alternates between 'doing' and 'doing nothing'. In other words, sometimes caring involves taking some form of action, and at other times standing back and allowing the service user to take responsibility for her- or himself. The carer will alternate between these two positions within the wider context of what went before and after the event itself. For Swanson (1991), this is characterised as enabling the service user to move towards self-care.

Mayeroff (1971) describes the purpose of caring as helping another to grow and self-actualise. Perhaps then, the object of caring in health and social care is to enable the service user to self-actualise and become self-caring. Linked to this is the focus of caring on the future. Mayeroff suggests that hope does not derive from dissatisfaction with the present compared to future possibility, but rather a belief that the plenitude of the present makes future growth a possibility. Swanson (1991) describes this as 'maintaining belief' and discusses the hope-filled attitude of the professionals who offer realistic optimism and belief in the service user's capacity to face whatever the future holds. In doing this, the caring relationship is one of trust; not the trust the service user has in the professional, but the trust the professional must have that the service user can make autonomous choices (Mayeroff, 1971).

If the goal of caring is to help another to achieve self-actualisation, there must be a relationship between the professional and the service user. This has been described in various ways. For example, Roach (1987) suggests that 'compassion' within caring involves sharing in the world of the service user, and 'commitment' includes devotion to the needs of others. Swanson (1991) describes 'being with' as being emotionally there with the service user whether physically there or not. Watson (1997: 54, 60), who equates caring with 'the heart and soul of nursing', adds another dimension – spirituality – when she describes the art of caring as 'soul to soul connecting'.

Whether or not one accepts the existence of a spiritual dimension to life, for Noddings (2003), the relationship between the professional and the service user is fundamental to the analysis of what caring is. She argues that whilst the relationship is not equal, and there is no agreement that it will be reciprocal, it is nevertheless the response of the service user that enhances or diminishes the caring relationship. For example, she suggests that the service user may respond in a positive way or the professional may be held off or ignored. If the service user refuses to take on the role of being cared for, then, it is argued, caring cannot happen.

Mayeroff (1971) however presents a different perspective. He suggests that there are one-sided caring relationships. The example he uses is that of a therapist caring for a service user. He argues that when the service user becomes able to care for himself, and could therefore conceivably care for the therapist, the therapeutic relationship ends. This recognition of the importance of maintaining professional relationships (General Medical Council, 2006) and the acknowledgement of boundaries to professional relationships (General Social Care Council, 2002; Nursing and Midwifery Council, 2008) ensures that a reciprocal caring relationship cannot develop between the health or social care professional and the service user.

Box 3.2   Definitions of art

Encarta (2009)

- the creation of beautiful or thought-provoking works
- beautiful or thought-provoking works produced through creative activity
- creation by human endeavour rather than by nature
- the set of techniques used by somebody in a particular field, or the use of those techniques
- the skill or ability to do something well.

Cambridge Advanced Learner's Dictionary (2009)

- the making of objects, images, music, etc. that are beautiful or that express feelings
- an activity through which people express particular ideas
- a skill or special ability.

Dictionary definitions suggest that art is both a process and a product (Box 3.2). Plato (c. 428–347 BC cited in Harrison-Barbet, 1990) asserted that art is the things which are acquired or produced by craft of skill, and Dr Johnson (cited in Crystal, 1990: 73) suggested that art is 'the power of doing something not taught by nature or instinct; as to walk is natural, to dance is art'. This all points to art being a skill or craft which is not instinctual, but is learned and directed towards the aesthetic and the expression of emotions. Harrison-Barbet (1990) thus asks whether there may be criteria that must be fulfilled for something to be considered art, or whether it may simply be a matter of subjective opinion; and if there are criteria, does the art of caring fulfil them? Consider again Vignette 3.4.

We all think we know an uncaring health or social care professional when we see one and we do not need a battery of empirical tests and carefully designed research projects to 'prove' it. As experienced professionals, we think we know when we are doing a good job, when an interaction is going well, or when a student is honing and developing new skills under our supervision. The question is: do we really think at all? There is a danger that work, even caring work, can become habitual, with a disregard for another's viewpoint. Do we treat others as we would like to be treated? Did Mary's doctor know that his humour was perceived as ill-meant? True caring has to include accepting that others do not necessarily want to be treated the way we want to be treated. People have different pain thresholds, different coping abilities, and of course different senses of humour. Thus, the question is whether science alone can provide the understanding of caring that health and social care professionals need in order to fulfil their role. With this in mind, we now examine caring in light of the philosophy of art.

The philosophy of art seeks to establish what it is that makes something into art. Are there criteria that must be fulfilled for something to be considered art, or is it a matter of subjective opinion? Harrison-Barbet (1990) poses this question by suggesting a comparison between the music of the Beatles and Beethoven, or the writing of a Mills and Boon novelist and Tolstoy. Which of these could be considered an expression of art, or are they all art carrying degrees of artistic value? He goes on to suggest that in philosophical enquiry into the nature of art, there are several areas for discussion. They include the purpose of art and issues related to beauty and judgement.

One area of enquiry in the philosophy of art is the question: what is the purpose of art? Sheppard (1987) suggests three potential purposes of art:

- *Imitation* or, in its widest sense, representation. This aims to provide a bridge between eternal ideas and the way in which they are sensed by the individual. Thus, the idea of beauty may be represented by music, painting or dance. Likewise, the activities of a health or social care professional could be a representation of the idea of caring. Another way of looking at it is to suggest that a painting of an elephant, for example, is a representation of an elephant – it is not the real thing but can be recognised as an elephant nevertheless, and a 'good' painting of an elephant will be able to represent the power and grace of an elephant as well as its physical form. Likewise, good physiotherapy would represent not just the ability to manipulate the human body, but to use touch in a way that represents caring.
- *Expression* which in art involves the communication of emotions. For example, the artist might communicate love by writing a poem and the painter might communicate sadness by painting a portrait of a tearful person. The difficulty with this view of art is that individuals have different emotional responses to the same stimuli, as is evident in the comments of different art critics to the same piece of work. Indeed, the example of Mary's response to the doctor's attempt at humour during cannulation is an example of this.
- *Aesthetic form* which is defined in terms of its effect, as the ability to arouse aesthetic emotion. Form is the way in which the elements – lines, colours, words, musical notes and so on – are arranged and fused into a complex unity. This is the creative aspect of art, the whole being more than the sum of the elements. It is only when the whole is viewed that it arouses aesthetic emotion. Form differs from expression in that in form the intention is to elicit emotion in the audience whereas in expression it is the artist's intention to communicate his or her own emotion. The artist may aim to arouse the aesthetic emotion by creating something beautiful, however the opposite is also applicable.

The audience gets a sense of what is beautiful by perceiving ugliness. This is one reason why works such as Damien Hirst's (2005) 'Prodigal Son (Divided)', a sculpture of a dead calf cut in half and suspended in formaldehyde, comes to be recognised as art.

If caring is to be considered an art, then presumably it must fulfil the purpose of art.

Vignette 3.5

I could see the nurse at the door of my room. I had just got my baby son off to sleep after a disturbed night of many medical tests. I was desperate that he was not woken again. But she was clearly coming in. I was surprised at how quietly she opened the door, she looked at my baby, then over to me and mouthed 'are you OK?'. I nodded and somehow I trusted her. She stood over my baby, just looking for a moment or two, then as she left the room she beckoned me to follow. Outside she quietly explained that she must check his vital signs as his temperature had been high earlier. I had to agree. We crept back into the room. First she quietly put her hand through the bars of the cot and held my baby's wrist. Then she silently and slowly lifted the heavy cot side, supporting the catch with her knee to stop it clanking. She lowered it and slowly moved the sheet aside. She gently placed the thermometer under my naked son's arm. He stirred but she put her hand gently on his back. It seemed a long wait but eventually she removed the thermometer. She put the cot-side up as cautiously as she had lowered it, all the time looking at my baby, then she put the thermometer away and wrote on the chart. She showed me what she had written, gave me the thumbs up, and left the room. It was awesome to watch her skills. I would have trusted my baby's life to her because she cared the way I did.

In this story, perhaps the concept the nurse was imitating or representing through her actions was a mother's care because the mother did not have the knowledge and skill to monitor vital signs. The emotions she was expressing were empathy and humanism. The emotions this evoked in the mother were awe and trust. Of course, just because we can identify characteristics of art in an episode of professional care, this does not make caring into art, but it equally does not lead us to reject the notion of caring as an art form.

Another major area of enquiry in the philosophy of art is the issue of beauty and judgement, the question being, what constitutes 'good' art and 'bad' art?

Good art, it could be argued, is that which achieves its objective, for example successfully representing an idea and object, or which successfully expresses an emotion, or draws on the emotions of others. Bad art, on the other hand, would be that which makes representation, or fails to express emotion. Perhaps the doctor's humour in Vignette 3.4 was bad art because he failed to elicit the emotion he sought: laughter.

Gendron (1994) used the fascinating analogy of tapestry to explore artistic nursing activities which could equally be applied to care by any health or social care profession. She described the warp as contextual knowledge and skills, available resources and policies; and the weft as the creative pattern of care. She further described the warp as a background structure involving scientific facts, conceptual ideas, technical skills and the assessing, planning, implementing and evaluating skills components of the care professional. This background structure also incorporates a professional's mandate and role as designated by the professional body. The weft of care was defined as 'a creative pattern ... woven on the warp strings of constraints, knowledge and skills' (Gendron, 1994: 25). She suggested that art in caring evolves: it is not a calculated construction, and asserted that the aesthetic pattern is paramount in caring, suggesting that the weft has the qualities of balance, harmony, rhythm, tone and unity. She argued that one needs to match caring actions to the person being cared for by attuning to, and synchronising with, her or him, and that requires an intuitive grasp or whole understanding. 'The analogy of warp and weft can help nurses think about how a structured framework for practice is combined with creative, individualised care for each person – the essence of nursing art' (Gendron, 1994: 29). This idea is in opposition to the notion that caring is an art and therefore taught, not innate. It suggests that we demonstrate caring behaviour primarily as a result of the desire to help someone; to enable them to cope with their illness or social difficulty, or to recover fully and perhaps enjoy an increased level of wellness and quality of life. Motivation to care cannot be taught, nor can it be gained from empirical research projects. It can, however, be nurtured.

Brink (1993) uses the analogy of the artist to facilitate understanding of the relationship between the art and science of caring in nursing. This analogy could be applied to any health or social care professional. Like the artist, the health or social care professional has some inherent talent for caring which needs to be nurtured and perfected through practice. All artists need to know something about their art, thus health or social care professionals need to know about their professional role. Brink (1993: 145) defines the science of caring as its knowledge base: 'Just as a dancer or a painter needs to know the science behind the dance or painting, so too the nurse needs to know the science behind the artistry of nursing'. She reflects on the critical importance of science for the knowledge and appreciation of what has led to the need for professional care, how health or social care professionals have solved problems, and what explanations they have offered to underpin their caring behaviour or interventions. Vignette 3.6 illustrates how two nurses used their knowledge to care for a child, but one used her creativity to make it beautiful.

Vignette 3.6

My baby was asleep so I was looking around the ward watching what was happening. A little boy with a broken arm was brought back from theatre. He was crying for his mother who had gone off to have a quick lunch. The nurse who received him settled him into bed and then picked up the chart and asked him to squeeze her hand. I guessed she wanted to check if his fingers moved OK in the plaster. The child was clearly too distressed to respond so she didn't get anywhere and spoke more and more loudly, almost shouting above his crying. That nurse was then called to the desk and another nurse went to the little boy. She moved very close to him, stroked his head and reassured him that mummy would be back soon and had just gone for a sandwich. The boy seemed to understand and began to calm down. Then the nurse held both his hands and said that he could squeeze her hands as hard as he wanted. Then she pretended it hurt and praised how tight he could squeeze, he giggled. She did the medical check without the child even knowing she had done it, and she cheered him up into the bargain. It was lovely to watch.

Here we see an example of how the nurse clearly reflected on how she could apply the science of assessment of peripheral circulation to a child who was screaming.

The early work of three nurse theorists (Carper, 1978; Peplau, 1988; Watson, 1981) adds further to our understanding of caring as art. They were writing explicitly about nursing but as health care provision has evolved, such that the caring element of all health and social care professionals is now recognised as important, much of what they say could be applied more widely than to nursing alone.

Carper (1978) describes aesthetics: the art of nursing, as one of four patterns of knowing in nursing. Again, this could be applied to any health or social care profession. She describes aesthetic knowing as expressive and made visible through action to the service user who is transformed by it. Carper does not however suggest that aesthetic knowing equates with the theory of aesthetics in art, that is, the notion of beauty and the emotions thus evoked (Sheppard, 1987). Instead, she links it with empathy, 'the capacity for participating in or vicariously experiencing another's feelings' (Sheppard, 1987: 16). She does, however, suggest that through aesthetic knowing, the design of nursing activities will have a sense of form and unity in the way in which they are structured, thus drawing implicitly on one of the concepts from the philosophy of art. Using this theory, the event described in Vignette 3.6 could be ascribed an aesthetic quality.

Watson (1981), in her discourse on nursing's scientific quest, made reference to art forms by suggesting that the motivation of both art and science is the same. She states that 'science is nothing else than the search to discover unity in the wild variety of nature or ... in the variety of our experiences. Poetry, painting, the arts are the same search ...' (Watson, 1981: 413). Thus, she argued that discoveries in science are a creation in the same way as original art. She went on to use this line of argument to support the use of humanistic research in nursing as a way of linking scientific rigor with the tradition of the art of nursing. Later, she makes the point that it is crucial to know the functions that science cannot perform for understanding professional practice in health care, and those that the humanities cannot perform in providing a knowledge base for a health care practitioner (Watson, 1985). She suggests that 'science is concerned with methods, generalizations, and predictions' while the humanities 'look for individual differences and uniqueness'. 'Science and the Arts each have their own value system and every individual practitioner has to relate to both of these while taking account of his or her own values' (Watson, 1985: 4).

Peplau (1988) makes more explicit reference to the philosophy of art. She suggests that nursing is an enabling, empowering, transforming art which has the aim of moving people in the same way that they may be moved by music or literature. She suggests that the medium of nursing art is the nurse herself, the process is in nurse–service user interactions, and the outcome is change which is within the service user and highly private. This view of nursing art in some ways relates closely to other art forms. For example, in painting, the medium is paint on canvas, the interaction is between the artist, the paint and the canvas, and the outcome is a painting which elicits individual and private emotions from each observer. An area where nursing does not equate with other art forms in Peplau's explanation is that there is a medium other than the artist in art. For painting, it is the paint; in music, it is the musical instruments; in poetry, it is language. Peplau does not identify any medium other than the artist in nursing as art. Also, Peplau fails to explore the elements from which a work of art is created. Nevertheless, this analogy of nursing and art adds to the notion of caring being more than purely a learned skill.

Stecker (1993) suggests that one of the modern views of the nature of art is that it is an open-ended concept and thus holds no essential attributes; there is merely family resemblance between art forms. This suggests that as caring does carry some of the characteristics of art, it can legitimately be described as the art of caring. The art, it seems, is the way in which evidence for practice is mediated to the service user. Health and social care professionals use knowledge from science and their own creativity to provide care suited to each individual service user.

This discussion of caring in relation to the philosophy of art offers an inclusive view of what constitutes evidence for practice, and should reduce the temptation to see knowledge as arising from either science or the humanities. Writing of caring in nursing, Seymour et al. (2003: 290) say: 'If research is presented solely as a scientific pursuit, then nurses will find it incongruent with their practice'. This suggests that both the art of caring and the scientific knowledge base need to inform the education of health and social care professionals. Skills such as critical thinking and critical appraisal need to be combined with caring characteristics such as compassion and respect for others. Similarly, the altruism that urges health and social care professionals to care creatively for individuals lacks value if it is not informed by the scientific knowledge necessary to provide the best possible care.

In a study of the meaning of caring to nurses in the intensive care setting, Wilkin and Slevin (2004) used semi-structured interviews with a sample of bedside nurses with data saturation being reached after 12 interviews. Content analysis using phenomenological methodology generated three themes:

- knowledge: knowing the patient, caring for significant others, technology, prioritising care, critical situations
- skills: nurse–patient interaction, physical support, advocacy, barriers to caring
- feelings: comfort, touch, empathy, presence, dignity, holistic care, caring for the carers.

Knowledge and skills are clearly the science element of caring and feelings the aesthetic element. The inclusion of dignity as part of the art of caring echoes the view of service users in the study by Age Concern (2005) discussed earlier.

Dignity features prominently in the government strategy for health and social care provision, so much so that it has launched a Dignity in Care campaign (DH, 2009b), one of its actions being to raise awareness of dignity in care. In response, the Nursing and Midwifery Council (2009) issued guidance to nurses and midwives saying that the essence of caring for older people 'is about getting to know and value people as individuals through effective assessment, finding out how they want to be cared for from their perspective, and providing care which ensures that respect, dignity and fairness are maintained' (p. 6). Furthermore, the response from the Social Care Institute for Excellence (2009) was to issue guidance on dignity in care to all social care workers. In it, dignity has been described as identified dignity with four overlapping ideas:

- **Respect**, shown to you as a human being and as an individual, by others, and demonstrated by courtesy, good communication and taking time

- **Privacy**, in terms of personal space; modesty and privacy in personal care; and confidentiality of treatment and personal information

- **Self-esteem, self-worth, identity and a sense of oneself**, promoted by all the elements of dignity, but also by 'all the little things' – a clean and respectable appearance, pleasant environments – and by choice, and being listened to

- **Autonomy**, including freedom to act and freedom to decide, based on opportunities to participate, and clear, comprehensive information. (p. 48)

This issue is discussed more fully in Chapter 6 which addresses values and the service user. Suffice to say here, the respect for dignity is a key value for caring health and social care professionals.

One of the complex aspects of care is the consequences when we as individuals, professionals or as a community do not care. If caring is such a fundamental value for health and social care professionals, this issue cannot be avoided. For example, when we don't care, we resist responsibility; we resist the call to care as basic aspects of our being, and a basic value of our profession. In not caring, we arrive at alienation, refusing the moral imperative to create cooperative, mutually rewarding experiences (Brechin, 1998a). Woodward (1997) speculates that a reduction in altruistic values in society is identified as one possible cause, and another the goal of efficiency, so that in the rush to meet tangible targets, expressive caring is one of the casualties, in that it is unaccounted for in the budget allocation. Nyström, et al. (2003) describe these episodes as non-caring encounters (Vignette 3.7).

Vignette 3.7

'Sometimes I am puzzled when I am lying on a trolley in the corridor. The same nurses are running here and there carrying pieces of paper. I don't know if it is the same paper or not, I have never asked about anything. But I have been wondering a lot why they rarely speak to me. They never tell me what they have done to me. I don't know anything' (Nyström et al., 2003: 764).

The question of what makes for good care can be evaluated in terms of outcomes, for example success could mean a sick service user recovers, or someone achieves optimum health, or even that someone self-actualises. Or good care could be evaluated in terms of the process, for example what the service user felt about the care given, and whether he or she felt cared for. Brechin (1998b: 175) suggests that 'any attempt to define "good care" must be explicit about what the purpose of the care is assumed to be'. For the caring professions, this purpose must be to ensure that everyone has safe and effective evidence-based care, delivered to the same high quality, no matter who they are, where they live or whatever their social circumstances.

As we have seen, caring takes two forms: the behavioural or instrumental form which relies on competent technical ability, and the affective or expressive form which involves human relationships. Instrumental caring is about behaviour and the actions a person takes to look after someone, whilst the expressive form includes an emotional element that values the uniqueness of each human being as an individual. Whilst the former is crucial to the conduct of professional practice, it is the latter which makes a qualitative difference to how people experience care and is the cornerstone of values-based care.

References

Age Concern (2005) 'The business of caring', *London Age*, Summer: 2–3.

Appleton, J.V. and Cowley, S. (2008) 'Health visiting assessment under scrutiny: a case study of knowledge use during family health needs assessments', *International Journal of Nursing Studies*, 45: 682–96.

Arthur, D., Pang, S. and Wong, T. (2001) 'The effect of technology on the caring attributes of an international sample of nurses', *International Journal of Nursing Studies*, 38: 37–43.

Barker, P. (2000) 'Reflection on caring as a virtue ethic within an evidence-based culture', *International Journal of Nursing Studies*, 37: 329–36.

Benner, P. (1984) *From Novice to Expert: Excellence and Power in Cinical Nursing Practice*. Menlo Park, CA: Addison-Wesley.

Brechin, A. (1998a) 'Introduction', in A. Brechin, J. Walmsley, J. Katz and S. Peace (eds) *Care Matters, Concepts, Practices and Research in Health and Social Care*. London: Sage, pp. 1–11.

Brechin, A. (1998b) 'What makes for good care?', in A. Brechin, J. Walmsley, J. Katz and S. Peace (eds) *Care Matters, Concepts, Practices and Research in Health and Social Care*. London: Sage, pp.170–87.

Brilowski, G.A. and Wendler, M.C. (2005) 'An evolutionary concept analysis of caring', *Journal of Advanced Nursing*, 50(6): 641–50.

Brink, P.J. (1993) 'The art and science of nursing', *Western Journal of Nursing Research*, 15(2): 145–7.

Cambridge Advanced Learner's Dictionary (2009) http://dictionary.cambridge.org/define.asp?key=4112&dict=CALD [accessed 29 November 2009]

Carper, B. (1978) 'Fundamental patterns of knowing in nursing', *Advances in Nursing Science*, 1(1): 13–23.

Crystal, D. (ed.) (1990) *The Cambridge Encyclopaedia*. Cambridge: Cambridge University Press.

Corbin, J. (2008) 'Is caring a lost art in nursing?', *International Journal of Nursing Studies*, 45(2): 163–5.

Department of Health (DH) (2009a) *Social Care Workforce*. Available at: www.dh.gov.uk/en/SocialCare/Aboutthedirectorate/DH_080186 [accessed 29 November 2009]

Department of Health (DH) (2009b) *Dignity in Care Campaign*. Available at: www.dhcarenetworks.org.uk/dignityincare/DignityCareCampaign/ [accessed 29 November 2009]

DLA Piper (2008) *DLA Piper Series: The Twentieth Century: How it Looked and How it Felt*. Liverpool: Tate.

Dunlop, M.J. (1986) 'Is a science of caring possible?', *Journal of Advanced Nursing*, 11: 661–70.

Encarta (2009) *MSN*. Available at: http://uk.encarta.msn.com/dictionary_1861690154/art.html [accessed 29 November 2009]

Engster, D. (2007) *The Heart of Justice: Care Ethics and Political Theory*. Oxford: Oxford University Press.

Gendron, D. (1994) 'The tapestry of care', *Advances in Nursing Science*, 17(1): 25–30.

General Medical Council (2006) *Good Medical Practice*. London: General Medical Council.

General Social Care Council (2002) *Codes of Practice for Social Care Workers and Employers*. London: General Social Care Council.

Harrison-Barbet, A. (1990) *Mastering Philosophy*. London: Macmillan.

Hawthorne, D. and Yurkovich, N. (1995) 'Science, technology, caring and the professions: are they compatible?', *Journal of Advanced Nursing*, 21(6): 1087–91.

Hirst, D. (2005) *The Agony and the Ecstasy*. London: Electa Napoli.

Information Centre, The (2006) *Staff in the NHS 2005*. London: The Information Centre.

Kenny, N.P. (1997) 'Does good science make good medicine?', *Canadian Medical Association*, 157(1): 33–6.

Kyle, T.V. (1995) 'The concept of caring: a review of the literature', *Journal of Advanced Nursing*, 21(3): 506–14.

Little, J.M. (2002) 'Humanistic medicine or values-based medicine ... what's in a name?', *Medical Journal of Australia*, 177(6): 319–21.

Malterud, K. (2001) 'The art and science of clinical knowledge: evidence beyond measures and numbers', *The Lancet*, 358: 397–400.

Mayeroff, M. (1971) *On Caring*. New York: HarperPerennial.

Morse, J.M., Solberg, S.M., Neander, W.L., Bottorff, J.L. and Johnson, J.L. (1990) 'Concepts of caring and caring as a concept', *Advancing Nursing Science*, 13(1): 1–14.

Musk, A. (2004) 'Proficiency with technology and the expression of caring: can we reconcile these polarized views?', *International Journal for Human Caring*, 8(2): 13–20.

Nay, R. (2003) 'Evidence-based practice: does it benefit older people and gerontric nursing?', *Geriatric Nursing*, 24: 338–42.

Noddings, N. (2003) *Caring*, 2nd edition. Berkeley, CA: University of California Press.

Nursing and Midwifery Council (2008) *The Code: Standards of Conduct, Performance and Ethics for Nurses and Midwives*. London: NMC.

Nursing and Midwifery Council (2009) *Guidance for the Care of Older People*. London: NMC.

Nyström, M., Dahlberg, K. and Carlsson, G. (2003) 'Non-caring encounters at an emergency care unit – a life world hermeneutic analysis of an efficiency-driven organisation', *International Journal of Nursing Studies*, 40: 761–9.

Olsen, D. (2000) 'Editorial comment', *Nursing Ethics*, 7(6): 470–1.

Peplau, H.E. (1988) 'The art and science of nursing: similarities, differences and relations', *Nursing Science Quarterly*, 1(1): 8–15.

Quinney, D., Pearson, M. and Pursey, A. (1997) '"Care" in primary health care nursing', in R. Hugman, M. Peelo and K. Soothill (eds) *Concepts of Care*. London: Arnold, pp. 56–75.

Roach, S. (1987) *The Human Act of Caring: A Blueprint for the Health Professions*. Ottawa: Canadian Hospital Association.

Rolfe, G. (2009) 'Some further questions on the nature of caring', *International Journal of Nursing Studies*, 46(1): 143–5.

Sack, D.A. (2006) *The Science of Caring*. Conference paper. Available at: www.prenger.msites.org/News/NewsStory.aspx?guid=3a493297-bc0a-4ba5-b6d7-59bcabed9b6a [accessed 29 November 2009]

Seymour, B., Kinn, S. and Sutherland, N. (2003) 'Valuing both critical and creative thinking in clinical practice: narrowing the research-practice gap?', *Journal of Advanced Nursing*, 142(3): 288–96.

Sheppard, A. (1987) *Aesthetics: An introduction to Philosophy of Art*. Oxford: Oxford University Press.

Social Care Institute for Excellence (SCIE) (2007) *Guide 9: Implementing the Carers (Equal Opportunities) Act 2004*. London: SCIE.

Social Care Institute for Excellence (SCIE) (2009) *Guide 15: Dignity in Care*. London: SCIE.

Standing Commission on Carers (2009) *Report of the Standing Commission on Carers 2007–2009*. London: Standing Commission on Carers.

Stecker, R. (1993) 'Aesthetics', in L. McHenry and F. Adams (eds) *Reflections on Philosophy: Introductory Essays*, New York: St Martin's Press, pp. 103–19.

Sturgeon, D. (2008) 'Skills for caring: valuing knowledge of applied science in nursing', *British Journal of Nursing*, 17(5): 322–5.

Swanson, K.M. (1991) 'Empirical development of a middle-range theory of caring', *Nursing Research*, 40(3): 161–6.

Watson, J. (1981) 'Nursing's scientific quest', *Nursing Outlook*, 29(7): 413–16.

Watson, J. (1985) *Nursing: The Philosophy and Science of Caring*. Boulder, CO: Associated University Press.

Watson, J. (1997) 'Artistry of caring: heart and soul of nursing', in D. Marks-Maran and P. Rose (eds) *Reconstructing Nursing: Beyond Art and Science*. London: Baillière Tindall, pp. 54–62.

Wilkin, W. and Slevin, E. (2004) 'The meaning of caring to nurses: an investigation into the nature of caring work in an intensive care unit', *Issues in Clinical Nursing*, 13(1): 50–9.

Wolf, Z.R., Giardino, E.R., Osborne, P.A. and Ambrose, M.S. (1994) 'Dimensions of nurse caring', *Journal of Nursing Scholarship*, 26(2): 107–11.

Woodward, V.M. (1997) 'Professional caring: a contradiction in terms?', *Journal of Advanced Nursing*, 26: 999–1004.

4 Values of Reductionism and Values of Holism

Tom Mason, Pete Hinman, Ruth Sadik, Doreen Collyer, Neil Hosker and Adam Keen

Introduction

Many readers of this text may be concerned about what it is to be human in a world that is ever-changing, complex and dynamic – in short, what is the *human condition*? Part of being human, in evolutionary or developmental terms, involves attempting to understand where we fit as mere 'particles' within the wider universe and where the atoms fit within our own individual, sub-universal selves. In our search for this understanding, our 'gaze' has been drawn to the heavens (holism) (James, 1984) as well as to the depths of the Soul (reductionism) (Rosenberg, 2006). Although, for many of us, our search continues, we can begin to draw some tentative conclusions. In this chapter, we focus our attention on four interrelated concepts that contribute to our humanistic perspective of health care delivery: reductionism, holism, value and humanism.

Reductionism

Reductionism is an ancient philosophy dating back, at least, to the early Greeks. It is a procedure that we employ to attempt to understand how a domain works by analysing its constituent parts. Domains can be any area of study from the physical sciences such as objects, planets, geography and biology to the social sciences of human behaviour, customs, rites, rituals and so on. Domains also traverse the philosophical sciences such as law, language and theology. In simple terms, we can apply reductionist procedures to the human body and, thus, arrive at an understanding of how the individual parts, for example the nervous system, alimentary system and endocrine system may function to maintain the integrity of the body in a state of what we know as 'life'. Through modern technology, we can deconstruct the human body down to minute structures with electromagnetic microscopy and theorise about molecular interaction (Ideker and Sharan, 2008). Furthermore, during this procedure of reductionism through all levels, including the universe, the world, the human body, the nervous system, neurones, synaptic gaps, chemicals and atomic structures, it is said that each smaller theory is absorbed into the greater. Given that we have only used the one example of the nervous system, if this were applied to all domains, across all sciences, then all theories could ultimately be absorbed into a 'global thesis' or a 'theory of everything' (Hawking, 1995). However, there may be problems with reductionism.

Holism

Holism dates back at least to the early Greeks and was summarised in the *Metaphysics* by Aristotle as the whole being more than the sum of its parts (Aristotle, 1998). The idea of holism, which is often said to be the opposite of reductionism, is that the properties or parts of an overall system cannot be totally understood by its components alone. If we take an example from physics, we might be able to understand how an engine works from an appreciation of its constituent parts, but we need another form of thinking to appreciate what it is to have a car, to understand the transport system and to appreciate our contribution to pollution and global warming. Thus, holistically, the human being is more than the sum of its component atoms, molecules, cells, organs, systems and body and would embrace aspirations, drives, ambitions, beliefs, social interactions and so on. In scientific holism, it is argued that because the whole is greater than the sum of its parts, then the overall behaviour of the system cannot always be predicted and leads to higher levels of complexity. An example of this can be seen in meteorology and the weather. This notion of multifaceted interaction is referred to in systems theory, chaos theory and complexity theory and, we would argue, is resonant in human nature.

What we value

Values operate as standards by which our actions are selected. There is little agreement in the science of values. Psychologists, sociologists, anthropologists and philosophers all disagree as to the emergence, function and dynamics of values (Giddens, 1997). However, at an axiomatic level, we understand values to be part of our societal traditions, mores, beliefs and normative prescriptions that bind communities together. This is despite the fact that they may be different in differing sub-groups of a community, may change over time, are affected by circumstances and may be held rigidly or weakly. In terms of health and social care, we can note that values are held in relation to reductionist approaches to understanding how the body works and holistic approaches in relation to the bio-psycho-socio-spiritual functioning of the self in the world. These contrasting approaches are often complementary in our understanding of health and social care and most assuredly are inter-related in the human condition.

Humanism

For most of us, when the integrity of the body or mind is threatened through being in a state of ill health or social difficulty, there is an underpinning drive to return to a state of health equilibrium and in doing so we may draw on numerous humanistic qualities (Herrick, 2005). We may ascribe whole-heartedly to a reductionist approach in the rationalist notion of cause and effect or we may draw on a holistic belief system in the mystical sense of being greater than the sum of our parts. In the former, we may rely, for example, on modern surgical or pharmacological remedies whilst in the latter we may draw on complementary therapies which remain largely unexplained. Furthermore, in this latter mode, we may rely on a greater authority by invoking a more divine therapeutic involvement through spirituality. In any event, we can see the human impact of all modes of thinking in the human condition.

   In this chapter, we will offer a critique of the contemporary reliance on evidence-based practice in Western health care systems and argue that this mode of thinking is merely one in a range of 'sciences'. It is our view that by focusing on a reductionist perspective alone merely eradicates the human-ness in health and social care, and that other modes of beliefs are *complementary* to the human condition.

The Nature of Value

Personal values are acquired and developed early on in our lives, shaping and influencing our thinking and behaviour (Warne and McAndrew, 2008). In relation to the bio-psycho-socio-spiritual functioning of the self in the world, values are neither identical with nor reducible to particular psychological phenomena: liking or disliking, preferring, evaluating, valuing or devaluing, whether taken singly or in various combinations (Lemos, 1995). By their individual disposition, personal values may never be articulated or shared. They indicate a belonging to different social groupings with a degree of homogeneity, such as our work, leisure activities or religious observance; they may or may not separate each grouping from others. Thus, heterogeneous groups with individual members with conflicting values may or may not be disclosed.

Taking the view that it is false to assume that people know what their values are, identifying one's values requires a person to decisively penetrate their moral index and form a values inventory. In reality, most people are living the values of others. Only when undertaking this conscious process and developing an inventory of personal values, identifying why these values are important to oneself and committing to them, are we able to live our own values. This exercise potentially reveals the ethical position of oneself and potentially the depth of self-indulgence or more sinisterly the extent of our immoral values. This account will incorporate a number of axiological studies and encompassing concepts which may include personal, organisational and societal notions of value and which also have correlated ethical and aesthetic features. These in turn will provide a distinct viewpoint on the nature of value and its influence on the human condition.

Values can constitute an individual's identity and also be shared by groups of different individuals, and similar individuals in a broader societal and cultural order. Examples could be respect for others, justice, concern for others, self-discipline, loyalty, competence and cooperation. Societal values could include authority, equality, legal protection and education. Social groups generally have a set of values, held within a loose psycho-social framework, for example religious or patriotic beliefs. Yet an individual's value of one concept may conflict or compete with another, creating a dissonance within that individual as shown in Vignette 4.1.

Vignette 4.1

My name is Pavel, I am a 54-year-old lorry driver, married with two young daughters, aged 9 and 11 years. I am in hospital with bad pain in my left leg. I am waiting for amputation due to insufficient blood supply caused partly by my smoking. Medication only dulls the pain and in an attempt to feel relaxed, I need to go out from the ward to smoke and the nearest place is the vestibule of the main

(Continued)

An elementary evaluation of the scenario could be that Pavel wants to smoke to help him relax from the sustained pain in his leg (the value of autonomy). Yet, he is aware that people using the main entrance will directly be affected by him smoking in a public area (maintaining the value of non-malfeasance). Continuing to smoke, he could exacerbate his symptoms and potentially affect his chances of continuing to work to maintain an income for his family (again, the value of non-malfeasance). In this case, the locus of control on what individually is viewed as the more respected value or values at a given time, is internally deliberated by Pavel (autonomy versus non-malfeasance). He views the use of smoking as his means of coping whilst in an acute stage of his condition. It could be claimed controversially by those accessing the hospital that his actions are universally harmful and antagonistic (malicious); also, from an emotive position, that he is jeopardising his employment status and the means to support his family (self-determination). Further, discarding the lit cigarette into a general waste bin or onto the carpeted floor in the main entrance as a careless act graphically illustrates the position Pavel selfishly takes. Taking an extreme view that there exists an increased risk of fire which could affect staff, service users and visitors, Pavel may fleetingly acknowledge his behaviour as an irresponsible act. Would he then excuse it by admitting that he was preoccupied by the pain in his leg, the prospect of his worsening health or the possibility of losing his job? Arguably, he had the choice of two courses of action, both of which he could view as morally right, but only one choice to make, a classic ethical dilemma (Purtilo, 1993). His choosing to take one course of action upholds his values at that time, though compromises and challenges the values of another (Beauchamp and Childress, 1994).

Which of those values should override the other? Is it the true nature of a human being to act in their personal interests first, and then respond altruistically when publicly exposed? Ethics can be defined as thinking and reasoning about morality (Rowson, 1990: 3), though it is also about being human and living in today's world: acknowledging that people have different views, values and experiences. Tschudin and Marks-Maran (1993: 3) suggest the view that 'it is not a question of who is right or wrong, but of how you can

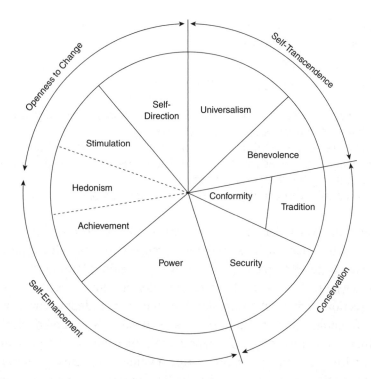

Figure 4.1   Guiding principles for life (Schwartz, 1992, 1994)

know what you believe is valuable, and stand by that value, and respect other people's values'. Further, they add that it is 'about understanding how your feelings and society's norms relate to each other, and how you decide for yourself and others'.

Although a powerfully influential and diverse concept, the nature of value, controversially, could be viewed as almost indeterminate. Furthermore, when value is described, an assumption is that it provides only a vague indication of its universal worth. If we take the view of Frankl (cited in Wirth, 2007), there are three central values in life: the experiential, or that which happens to us; the creative, or that which we bring into existence; and the attitudinal, or our response in difficult or challenging circumstances. Employing all three simultaneously in our activities is ultimately how we thrive as human beings, both altruistically and egocentrically, with competing beliefs.

Schwartz (1992, 1994) used his 'Schwartz Value Inventory' (SVI) for a wide survey of over 60,000 people to identify common values that acted as guiding principles for their lives, depicted here as a circular representation of the value types (Figure 4.1). The value type domains are 'super grouped' into four higher-order value types: on one side, 'openness to change' and 'self-enhancement'; on the opposite side of the circle, 'conservation' and 'self-transcendence'. On examination, the values form something of a spectrum with successive values often having a close relationship.

Described in detail within his published work (1992, 1994), Schwartz's domains of his inventory include following value types:

- 'power' – those individuals that value social status, prestige and dominance over people and resources
- 'achievement' – relating to personal success and admiration
- (benevolence) – advocating an ethical virtue of non-malfeasance, promoting the welfare of others
- 'tradition' – representing a respect of traditions and customs.

Other value types identified by Schwartz et al. (2002) reveal more indulgent characteristics, such as 'hedonism' representing a value type where preference is given to pleasure and self-gratification; 'stimulation' representing a group of values that express a preference for an exciting life; and 'self-direction', a distinct group of values that value independence, creativity and freedom. Along with more principled value types noted within the inventory, is a 'conformity' value type containing values that represent obedience, with 'universalism' representing a value type whose preference is for social justice and tolerance, and, finally, 'security' as a value orientation containing values relating to the safety, harmony and welfare of society and of oneself. It could be argued that exposure to the value types endorsed by Schwartz et al. (2002), as elements of our moral index, will enhance the development of oneself. We grow from infancy, learning and rehearsing, executing learned behaviours, employing numerous value dimensions. These signify our status as an individual along with a profound set of psychosociological and spiritual principles, be they inhibited by custom or expressed creatively without bounds. By tacit adherence to one's own value code, it is the expression of oneself.

Return to Task Orientation

From value to task

In the reductionist ideology, there is a tendency to focus on the individual part, which has the potential for the overall picture to become confused. For example, in the development of the industrialised world, in relation to the modes of production, factories were designed for individuals to work on one small component of an overall product. This mechanistic approach ensured the effective use of labour, but at a cost of tedium for the workers. Employees working on a conveyor-belt production line may have the reductionist task of putting a particular bolt on a specific part of the construction but the overall end-product of a car, for example, is merely a distant figment. Throughout the last century, this conveyor-belt industrialisation became known as Ford-ism, after the Ford factory production of cars, with its focus on task orienta-tion, efficient modes of production (at a physical and psychological cost to the workers) and consumerism (Bakker and Miller, 1996; Lundy, 2007). It is not surprising that in the post-Second World War era and the inception of the NHS in the UK, the medical model and numerous nursing models were reductionist in nature, viewing parts of the body and mind as 'broken' and requiring health services to 'fix' them (Shaw and Mountain, 2007). This mechanistic approach to health care saw hospitals as factories with input, throughput and output recorded as admission rates (Richman, 1987). This led to a concentration on the human being as a set of sub-components that if all are working effectively constitutes the overall state of being human. Unfortunately (or fortunately), this falls short of understanding the essence of *being* human (Norman, 2004).

Throughout the closing decades of the last century, and the early part of this century, two major factors have converged to influence our current health and social care services. These factors are technological advancements and political ideologies. The development of the microchip has led to the huge leap forward in information technologies with giant strides being made in health science. This, Foucault (1973) suggests, has produced a 'medical gaze' on the micro-aspects of the body with keyhole surgery, fibre-optics and map-ping techniques revealing the previously hidden parts of the body as visible entities on TV screens. Whilst progression of health science is creditable and welcome, it comes at a potential cost to the service user at an individual level. The increase in technology, for all health care professionals, can lead to a focus on equipment rather than on the service user (Cooper, 1993). By neces-sity, complicated equipment requires careful and expert management, which centres the attention on the task at hand. The task, or job, is to ensure the effective functioning and operation of the technology rather than the serv-ice user. This has been noted in numerous health care arenas (Heath et al., 2003; Smith, 1997).

The second factor or, more accurately, the second set of factors, involves political ideologies. The consumerist approaches within the capitalism of Margaret Thatcher and the Conservative government of the 1980s and 1990s led to many health and social care reforms being set within a market-economy-driven structure. The values of care delivery were subsumed within the dominant force of profit. The drive for profit inevitably involves competition and the use of cheap labour. Although ideologically such a consumerist approach in businesses would suggest the evolution of waste reduction and increased quality of services, in health and social care organisations, these drives may well be misdirected (Smith, 1997). An example would be the placing of hospital cleaning services with private companies, who competed for the contracts in the open market. This resulted, as would be expected, in the use of cheap labour and cleaning materials, at a reduced cost to the company with the consequences of a poor cleaning service (Cooper et al., 2003). Some have suggested that the result of this is the high levels of infections (the Superbugs – MRSA, C. Diff.) seen in some of our contemporary hospitals (Greenstein et al., 2003). Over the past decade, New Labour policies have fared little better with Foundation Trusts and the implementation of the Modern Matron having little impact (Bolton, 2003). Although Tony Blair attempted to re-focus attention on the individual service user, the government appeared to lose sight of the holism of the person through an emphasis, even obsession, on quantifying the entire process of health and social care delivery. Indeed, there has also been the suggestion of measuring how much compassion a nurse shows and how often they smile at service users! (Carvel, 2008).

Tensions in health and social care

Emerging from the foregoing brief history of contemporary health and social care influences are a number of themes and these are: expectations, roles and accountability. Expectations refer to what can be realistically anticipated from health and social care services in relation to the limitations in resources and professional knowledge (Manser and Staender, 2005). For example, there is frequent debate concerning the expensive price of certain drugs and a care provider's decision not to provide it on the NHS for individual service users suffering from cancer. Furthermore, we appreciate that despite modern treatments, service users continue to die, thus indicating the limits to medicine (Illich, 1976). However, expectations also involve the prediction of standards as a norm to be anticipated. In this sense, it is what we can expect from a service after we have balanced the tension between limitations and desires. Another tension involves the changing role dynamics of the professionals, the service users and their families. From the traditional accepted abdication of responsibility within the Parsonian sick role (Parsons, 1951), service users now share accountability for their illness or social situation, are partly responsible for recovery and are expected to contribute to their care (Fendrick et al., 2001; Holden, 2007). Professional roles have changed in response to the dynamic of contemporary health and social care services with a strong emphasis on the effective management of the infrastructure of the organisation. At a macro-organisational level, this focuses on waiting times, bed management, early discharge, case closure and so on, and at a micro-organisational level on care plans, birth plans, administrative forms and so on. Relatives' roles have also changed as they expect the care services to function like any other service. Complaints have increased as the silent respect for professionals, particularly doctors and nurses, has evaporated (Blickstein, 2007; Cowan and Anthony, 2008; Floyd, 2008). It would appear that they are now just as likely to be threatened as thanked. Accountability has emerged as a powerful factor in modern health and social care with increases in litigation, compensation and out-of-court settlements (Blickstein, 2007; Floyd, 2008). The setting of targets by the government has allowed for the monitoring of results with the corollary of dismissal in the event of failure (Shaw et al., 2008). These factors, then, have coalesced to change the value structure within health and social care which encourages a focus on the reductionist parts and loses sight of the service user at a holistic level.

A few examples should now suffice to bring these factors into stark relief. Service users are expected to comply with the professionals' request for early self-help and discharge. They are also expected to negotiate care and contribute through becoming autonomous. Relatives are now expected to be more fully involved in the service users' care, for example in cooking and feeding, toileting, washing, cleaning and shopping. The move towards a closer relative involvement is reflected in partners attending childbirth, parents staying with their children in hospital over the 24-hour period and families being involved in the single assessment process for vulnerable people in the community. Professionals may shed these interactional and interpersonal aspects of care delivery as they expect service users and relatives to manage these holistic elements. If relatives are expected to provide this, then it allows the professionals to focus more on the management and operationalising aspects of the task.

Seen in reductionist terms, task allocation is managed through assessing the requirements of the task (what needs to be done), operationalising it (doing it) and evaluating the outcome (reflecting on it) (Pearcey, 2007). However, the skills and competencies required to undertake task management – even a health or social care task – may not be those required by a holistic professional. It may be that a manager has the skills of task allocation whilst the health or social care professional has the skills to perceive the service user in a holistic manner. In nursing, for example, the care role has come under scrutiny in recent times in relation to the skills and competencies that are required (Pearcey, 2008). The current move in the UK to provide nursing education at degree level only would suggest that qualified nurses will be a minority of the health care workforce in the future. The main caring role will likely be undertaken by a larger group of unregistered Health Care Assistants (HCAs), a highly skilled but smaller nursing group and a service user population expected to meet their own health care needs (Bach et al., 2008). This phenomenon is also seen in other professional areas with roles such as physician's assistant and mental health worker developing. Vignette 4.2 illustrates the possible outcome for service users.

Vignette 4.2

Jim and Betty are both octogenarians, have been married for 63 years and have three children, the closest of whom lives 103 miles away. In order to assist Betty and Jim, a carer comes and showers Jim each morning. Early one morning Jim sustains a fall which results in admission to hospital after sustaining a fractured femur and cuts to his head and legs. He also has dementia which is made worse by unfamiliar surroundings. Betty accompanies Jim on his admission at 03.30 hours and as he is proving difficult to manage, chronic staff shortages and the fact that Betty and Jim have never spent a night apart, the staff encourage Betty to remain in a side room with her husband. The following morning a Healthcare Support Worker (HSW) arrives and presents Betty with a bowl in order to assist her husband with his hygiene. At 15.00 hours a Staff Nurse goes to check on Jim and finds him and his wife collapsed, surrounded by untouched breakfast and lunch trays.

The questions that should arise from this are twofold. First, would the outcomes of the scenario change if on admission there had been no chronic staff shortage? This is debatable given that the full staff complement would have predominantly been Healthcare Support Workers (HSWs), Second, if a qualified nurse had gone in with the bowl as opposed to the HSW, would she have noted that Betty appeared exhausted and had not been able to get a drink?

Structured Assessment

Plato deals with the notion of learning in his inimitable fashion within the Socratic dialogue *Meno* (Hutchinson, 1997) and this has an interesting perspective on the idea of 'assessment'. Meno begins by asking Socrates to explain to him whether virtue is acquired by teaching or by practice; or if neither ... then whether it comes to man by nature, or in what other way? The answer involves issues of education, learning and teaching within the overarching concept of what constitutes knowledge. To facilitate Socrates' point, he invites a young slave boy over who represents ignorance and the uneducated in early Greek times. Socrates then asks the slave boy to draw a square in the sand and, through a series of questions and answers, leads the boy through some complex geometric examples dealing with squared numbers and angles. At the end of the session, he then sends the slave boy off to his work and turns to Meno to enquire whether the slave boy has learnt anything, is now educated or if the knowledge was always there and just needed to be brought out. A lengthy discussion takes place regarding the process of what had happened in the interaction between Socrates and the slave boy. What is relevant to us here is the issue that we do not actually know whether the slave boy is educated or not or has learnt anything from Socrates because he is not assessed, and he never returns in the dialogue to give any other indication, practical or theoretical, that he has learnt something. All we have to go on is the answers he gave to Socrates' questions when asked.

However, what is clear within the Meno dialogue is the ongoing formative assessment as Socrates continually gauges whether the boy understands as he does, indeed, frequently claim to do so. However, without a summative assessment, we do not actually know whether the value of the knowledge, education and learning is applied, either in practice or in theory. From this, we make an assumption that it would be a positive endeavour if we could assess the slave boy to see if he had learnt something. We could undertake this assessment through a number of formal instruments by examinations, assignments and projects, for example, or we could employ a structured evaluation by observing a practical test in which he would do a task to reveal his knowledge of geometry. Of course, we juxtapose this type of formal assessment with a more intuitive evaluation which would incorporate watching and listening to the interaction between Socrates and the slave boy with a belief in the *process* of the educational framework, in this case questioning and answer. The issue now turns to the underpinning values inherent in both formal and informal (or intuitive) assessments.

Formal and intuitive assessments

In contemporary health and social care, there is an emphasis on evidence-based practice and this is as much the case in the practice arena as it is in professional education itself. There is a reliance on the structured assessments that are considered to be scientific in the sense that they usually involve some degree of measurement. The growth in instruments to perform a degree of assessment is vast and continues to expand (Mason and Whitehead, 2003). This reliance on quantification reflects the belief in the hard science of numbers with statistics being the favoured religion. In clinical terms, there are APGAR scores at birth (Finster and Wood, 2005), percentiles through growth (Hemachandra et al., 2007), measures of quality of life (Rajmil et al., 2004) and all manner of scales of mental health, personality function, behavioural repertoires and the experience of pain (Williamson and Hoggart, 2005), to mention but a few. In professional education, we are familiar with unseen examinations, assignments, essays, objective, structured, clinical examinations, portfolios, multiple-choice exams and so on. In all these, the values pivot on the notion of hard evidence extracted by an array of measurement tools, some clearly quantitative but others most assuredly qualitative.

Informal, or intuitive, assessments, on the other hand, are held to be more strictly qualitative and by dint of this term are devalued in relation to the evidence-based approaches. However, a brief foray into this intuitive assessment procedure reveals a different picture. Intuition is an internal and often subconscious process that is grounded in tradition, experience and instinct. Traditional values are those that have been passed on from generation to generation and have been formulated in evolutionary terms over hundreds and thousands of years. They form the basis of our collective unconscious and make up our cultural mosaic, which as we can see contributes to establishing differences between societies. However, despite these differences, there are consistent imperatives across cultures, perhaps in varying strengths, but none the less inherently established, such as caring for the sick and socially deprived. Experience can be said to emanate from an interaction with traditional values and also contributes in turn to maintaining them. Once exposed to, say, the values of caring for others, we then employ that experience to perpetuate those beliefs for future generations and teach others those values. Experience of those principles becomes established as the normative standards by which our culture functions and certain behavioural actions become expected, such as caring for the sick. This type of experience becomes respected and valued. Instinct refers to innate patterns of behaviour that occur in response to certain stimuli without necessarily any actual experience of how to act in a certain way. This can be said to be a way of intuitively acting or thinking in a pre-determined and natural way. For example, if an egg is hatched in an incubator, the caged bird will grow and have the skills to build a nest independently of the experience of seeing one built. Therefore, the assumption is that we, as humans, may have certain values (in our example, caring for the sick), even if we were born and raised on an island away from all other humans. In short, we would instinctively value caring for others.

Dehumanisation

In philosophical terms, humanism refers to a number of interrelated concepts that are concerned with what it is to be a human being in this world. It involves the nature, defining characteristics, abilities, powers, education, culture and, most notably, the values of being human. Humanism is both a simple and a complex concept. In simple terms, it is about the recognition of the value of others and sharing this world in a common community in which everyone has an equal place. It is also concerned with the ability to have empathy, in which we recognise the pains and pleasures in others and reflect them back into ourselves. In this way, we can 'share' and 'know' others' feelings. However, humanism is also a complex, yet coherent, system of substantive, ontological, epistemological, anthropological, sociological and psychological perspectives. These bring in educational, aesthetic, political, ethical and moral claims, which contribute to the cultural mosaic that forms community structures (Kurtz, 2006; Norman, 2004).

There are, of course, many more aspects to being human and most writers on this topic would include spirituality, poetry, art, history and morality, to name but a few. Seeing such aspects to being human is clearly a reductionist approach, which sub-divides human nature into ever more micro components and suggests that each part is separate from the other. In reality, all aspects are interrelated and have a dynamic affect on each other, with each contributing to the holistic nature of being human (Herrick, 2005). When we think of the self, we predominantly think of what it is like to be 'me' and we perceive our 'self' in relation to the world from the 'I' that is within us. However, as we live in this world with others, it is our relation to others that makes us human and this relation is known as the 'I–Thou' primary relation, in the classic text by Buber (1937). Within the 'I–Thou' relationship with others, each culture, community and society arranges a set of social norms that govern how we are to behave towards each other. These norms prescribe our social action and take into account the nature of being human, which outlines ways of acting towards each other with accompanying sanctions when they are transgressed (Giddens, 2000).

Difference and distance

The role of norms in regard to dehumanisation is exemplified in the works of Szasz (1974), Bauman (1996) and McPhail (1999). According to Szasz, mental illness is traditionally based on the medical ethic that a neurological cause lies behind each variance from normal behaviour and thought. Yet, the judgement of 'normal' is based on a complex interplay of sociological, ethical and political factors and this, therefore, has the potential to dehumanise. In order to dehumanise, we must be able to establish a difference between 'them' and 'us' and this difference then carries some element of a devaluation towards 'them'. We are all aware of the many prejudices that occur around the world and we can name racial, religious and national as exemplars of such intolerances. Once such differences have been identified and devalued, we can then become detached from the commitment to the relationship with the 'other' and separate ourselves from empathy with them. 'They' become not like us and 'They' are thus distanced from us. However, before we turn our attention to health and social care issues, it is important to examine how we, as human beings, can now move beyond mere distancing of the 'other' to actually acting negatively towards them.

Bauman (1996), in his study of the Holocaust, describes how some social theorists compare the processes required for the implementation of the 'final solution' to those of modern enterprises and bureaucracy. This gives the historical nature of the Holocaust analysis a modern relevance, particularly in relation to health and social care. During the Holocaust, some 6 to 12 million people were put to death (Bauman, 1996). Whilst the starting point of the Holocaust required a devaluation and alienation of the learning disabled, the mentally ill, the Gypsies, the homosexuals and the Jews, the ultimate outcome required the application of efficient business processes, modern technology and systematic surveillance techniques. Those involved in the process were arguably distanced from the moral implications of their actions through the 'normality' imposed by the organisational process itself. In short, the process of elimination becomes 'normal'. Once the distance between 'them' and 'us' is established, 'they' have to all become the same. They become 'The Jew' (Lyotard, 1990). This is personified in the shaving of their heads and making them wear the same striped 'pyjamas' in order to maintain the detachment.

There are many examples of dehumanisation and the Holocaust is probably in the extreme. However, we must remember that it was men of medicine, having taken the Hippocratic Oath, that performed the medical experiments in the Holocaust. Furthermore, their defence at the Nuremburg trials was largely not based on a denial of their involvement but that the experiments were legal (Hitler had changed the law) and had peer review acceptance. However difficult it is to understand how medical professionals can break such a code of morality, we should note that such transgressions have been observed in 'normal' people. We should compare the Eugenics movement in the UK, which saw the hospitalisation of thousands of people with learning disabilities and mental health problems over the previous century and the analogy of the communist witch hunts in the USA. Both these show how 'normal' people may lose sight of the individual in an overarching prejudice of belief.

At the level of science, Milgram (1974) conducted a series of controversial experiments testing obedience (Blass, 2002). His experiments involved 'normal' subjects administering increasingly (perceived) painful electric shocks as a form of punishment to a distanced victim (the stooge). The results of the study showed that the various control mechanisms for moral agency can be disengaged in 'normal' people and that this disengagement is inversely correlated to the distance between the subject and the victim (Milgram, 1974). Haney et al. (1973) investigated the process of dehumanisation and de-individualisation in a controlled 'total environment'. The two-week experiment, known as the Stanford Prison Experiment, in which 24 college students were assigned the roles of either prisoner or guard, was disbanded after only six days as altered behaviour within the study sample evoked serious ethical concerns. It was shown that individuals, who had been previously psychometrically tested for their 'normality' could, when placed in certain contrived situations, adopt roles beyond the boundaries of their previous norms, laws, ethics and morals (Zimbardo et al., 1999).

The history of the Holocaust, therefore, demonstrates that dehumanisation can occur in people who are considered to be 'normal' and can take place in the monstrous event as well as the mundane of everyday life. In fact, it is quite surprising the extent to which it is occurring throughout our society – for example, in sport with the use of performance enhancement (Culbertson, 2007), in reality TV shows (Menon, 2006) and in the creation of the 'enemy-image' (Maiese, 2003). Therefore, it should come as no surprise to realise that in health and social care settings dehumanisation is also taking place.

Dehumanised values in health and social care

Health and social care settings are part of an overall system of services that form an industry of care. But, by the nature of the services that are delivered, they are usually constructed as large organisations. Here we will use hospitals as an example. Like most large organisations, they require systems of process to manage their productivity and these systems may well emerge to be the focus of scrutiny in themselves, rather than the product that they produce. When dealing with tangible products, such as motor cars, the systems that produce them can be quality assured in an effective and quantifiable way involving measures of performance-related outcomes. Furthermore, whilst the product of a good car is set within parameters of a quality assurance framework, a health condition transcends these boundaries to an existential level of meaning. In measuring a medical condition in terms of waiting times, inpatient admission rates, throughput and output, outcome data and discharge times, which are all necessary and appropriate, we can lose sight of the quality of that journey for the person concerned. The analogy of the construction of a car through the factory and the mechanistic process of reconstructing a human being through the hospital is, perhaps, a little hackneyed these days. However, it suffices to deliver the message that there is something beyond the human journey through ill health or social difficulty that modern health and social care services can miss if their focus is limited to these measures alone.

Concentration on outcomes, such as inpatient days, can evade issues of the lived experience of the quality of that inpatient time, and the meaning that it has in the more holistic life journey for that person. This is part of the dehumanisation process of modern health and social care services which can focus on the system processes and outcomes rather than the individuals within it. Whilst most of us are advocates of science and the production of evidence, it is within the system of health and social care that we must remain vigilant in protecting the values and morals that underpin it. In focusing on the body and its reductionist parts, we can lose sight of the person within the care system. There are obvious areas in the care services in which dehumanisation can occur. For example, it has been noted that the effective application of what is considered to be best evidence-based practice in Intensive Care Units can lead to dehumanisation, even by the very best of caring practitioners (Calne, 1994; Corrigan et al., 2007). In surgical procedures, cradled within modern notions of science, there is a danger of dehumanisation but, thankfully, also a call for surgeons not only to be *Homo sapiens* but *Homo moralis* too (Likhterman, 2005). The advancement of medical technology itself, implicitly accepted as a good thing, is also a warning against dehumanisation (Heath, et al., 2003) as is the encroachment of modern information systems (Keen, 2006). These warnings serve to remind us that the values that underpin health and social care are more important than the mere process of application, as illustrated in Vignette 4.3.

> ### Vignette 4.3
>
> Kelly, a 24-year-old woman with severe learning disabilities, was admitted to the Accident and Emergency Department claiming to have swallowed several batteries. She had done this on several other occasions. She was difficult to manage and aggressive when approached by staff. Debates ensued as to the best approach to gathering information about the size and number of batteries she had ingested but Kelly was not amenable to rational discussions. She was refusing any treatment and demanded to be allowed to go home. The decision of the team following discussions between the medics and the nursing staff was to allow her to go home.

Here, the rationale for the decision was that as she had learning disabilities, and that she had brought this upon herself, she would not be able to learn not to do it again, so did not warrant valuable resources. The staff did not consider a psychiatric referral or compulsory admission under the Mental Health Act but rather focused on the severity of the learning disabilities. Thus, the individualised values of humanism gave way to overarching problems of management and the limitations of resources. It could be argued that, because Kelly had learning disabilities, she needed more resources to help her than someone who fully understood what he or she was doing.

Medical Model and Complementary Therapies

Modes of knowledge

For the purpose of this discussion, there can be said to be three modes of knowledge (or ways of thinking) concerning the world in which we live (Nachmias and Nachmias, 1981). These modes of knowledge are:

- *Authoritarian*: in this mode, the focus is upon sapient knowledge that is espoused from a source that is considered wise, and there is little questioning as to its truth, accuracy or alternatives. This mode can best be described in parent–child terms when the authority of the mother and father announce to the toddler the pending arrival of a new baby brother or sister delivered by a Stork. At that stage, it is unquestionably accepted as true and accurate by the young child. Whilst we may like to believe that we grow out of this mode of thinking, and indeed many do, for some it remains into adult life and knowledge is accepted when authority figures issue dictums which are unquestioned. These 'authorities' may be, for example, religions (doctrine), political persuasions (the Party line) or medical knowledge ('the doctor said so').

- *Mystic*: this mode is concerned with a state of consciousness that is said to be in tune with a higher order of reality, and access to this knowledge is achieved through prophets, divines, gods, mediums, clairvoyants and parapsychologists, to name but a few. In this mystic mode, there is a belief in a link between supernatural authorities and the bio-psycho state of the individual. Thus, for example, we look to astrology to inform us as to the effects on our earthly lives. We can recognise a wide array of strands of mysticism in many traditions and cultures and it is a notably powerful theme in both Islamic and Buddhist philosophy. Superstitions are based in this mode as we believe certain behaviours may invoke higher-order interventions, such as walking under a ladder bringing bad luck. Behaviour enacted from this mystical mode of knowledge is difficult to change as it requires many refutations before it affects the individual's belief in the mode of thinking (Nachmias and Nachmias, 1981). An example is circumcision based on religious beliefs.

- *Rationalistic*: this mode is concerned with a philosophical belief in knowledge that is said to be gained through the process of logic. This process is based on two assumptions: first, that we can apprehend the world independently of the observed phenomena, and secondly that forms of knowledge exist prior to our experience of them. The cause-and-effect relationship is seen in isolation and understood as being independent of extraneous influences such as gods, prophets and devils. This mode of knowledge is known as the method of science and is held in high esteem in Western societies (Nachmias and Nachmias, 1981). For example, the perception that illnesses such as cancer or HIV are often related to behaviour such as smoking, drug abuse and sexual promiscuity results in less sympathy for sufferers, and demonisation of those who behave in these ways.

All three modes of knowledge can be seen independently but we can also note that there may be areas of overlap. In fact, there is nothing to negate a belief in all three modes at the same point in time. Numerous astronauts who walked upon the moon believed in the rationalistic mode of science through their knowledge of physics but also operated within the authoritarian and mystic modes through a belief that a divine being was safeguarding them on their journey (Nachmias and Nachmias, 1981).

The medical model

The medical model is a term that is widely employed but not well defined. Its basic premise is that it is focused on the physical aspects of the body, in terms of sickness and health, and the physical treatments that are available. This is based in the rationalistic mode of thinking in relation to the logic of cause and effect. However, it applies equally to issues of the mind, and to social situations where there is deemed to be an identifiable cause that leads to the situation the individual finds her- or himself to be in. The medical model assumes a power imbalance between doctor (or other care professional) and patient (or service user) with the former being the technical expert and the latter the passive recipient of services. Within this framework, the medical model attempts to explain disease or social difficulty by establishing its aetiology, its agent and its path of restoration. It views the person as a machine with reductionist parts that can be repaired. However, in viewing the person in these limited terms, it fails to appreciate the wider empirical diversity of the social and spiritual aspects of the human condition. Although the majority of Western medicine, and much of social care, is grounded in this model, there are some health and social care professionals who broaden their model to encompass the social and spiritual aspects, notably in the fields of mental health care. The notion of all medical models is underpinned by a process known as medicalisation.

The medicalisation process

The medicalisation process is concerned with how areas of life, or domains of the human condition, are brought within the framework of medicine. This is what Foucault (1973) called the medical 'gaze'. Examples of this 'gaze' include childbirth, child-rearing, bereavement and dying (Clark, 2002), these being domains of traditional life that would previously be encompassed by the village midwife, families and religious orders respectively, but are now part of 'medicine'. There are many other examples of this ever-encroaching 'gaze' in contemporary society, such as sexual behaviour (Hart and Wellings, 2002), misery (Pilgrim and Bentall, 1999) and rage (Fisher, 2006). The process by which this medicalisation occurs has five components:

- *Identification* – medicine must be able to establish a difference between normal and abnormal. It needs to know what constitutes normal (levels, functioning, behaviour, thoughts and so on) from which it can then establish someone who is operating outside the parameters of this normal. Thus, there is a need to identify the difference.
- *Classification* – once the difference is established, the 'condition' must be placed within a classification system which absorbs it into the theoretical structures of that particular nosological framework. Nosology is a branch of medicine that is concerned with classifying conditions according to whether they fit, for example, into physical systems such

as the nervous system, or psychiatric systems such as psychoses. Classification gives the impression of knowledge of the condition.

- *Diagnosis* – this is concerned with a concept beyond classification and involves providing an aetiological explanation. The medicalisation process involves providing clarification on how the condition arose, where it comes from, how it happened, etc.
- *Treatment* – for the medicalisation process to continue, a treatment intervention must be offered. This may be merely palliative in cases of terminal illness or abstract in psychiatric conditions. Nonetheless, an intervention must be both suggested and accepted, at least by some.
- *Prognosis* – to complete the process, a prediction is required as to the anticipated outcome following treatment. Forecasting the progress of the condition is an extension of the cause-and-effect logic of science. The prognosis does not necessarily require accuracy, it merely needs to be predicted.

It should be noted that if the process cannot be completed, then the 'condition' is not likely to be accepted within the medical model and, similarly, if an established medical condition becomes unsupported in any of the components of the medicalisation process, then it is likely to fall out of the medical frame of reference. An example of this is homosexuality which was considered a psychiatric condition up to the 1960s but then abandoned as a medical entity thereafter. A more recent example is the acceptance of myalgic encephalomyelitis (ME) which prior to total medicalisation was known as Chronic Fatigue Syndrome (ME Association, 2009).

Health beliefs and complementary medicine

Health belief models take many forms, both within and across cultural groups. Numerous distinctions can be drawn, including (a) supernatural and natural, (b) personalistic and natural, (c) retribution and justice and (d) internalising and externalising (Richman, 1987). In all these, causes of ill health are sought through all modes of knowledge: authoritarian, mystical and rationalistic. Health belief models range from cosmopolitan (rationalistic) approaches to traditional approaches, which vary across cultures. We do not have space to outline the numerous health belief models but one will suffice as an example. The American Navaho Indians may spend a quarter of their time involved in healing rites and 'to be cured means social reconciliation with kin, ancestors and nature. Treatment is family and community orientated therapy' (Richman, 1987: 20). Complementary medicine is a more modern term for 'alternative', 'marginal', 'fringe', 'quack' and 'traditional' and the array of approaches within the terms is immense. There is an attempt to portray cosmopolitan medicine as scientific, and traditional medicine as unscientific, and similarly terms such as 'orthodox' and 'unorthodox' have been applied as value judgements. The modes of thinking outlined above can also be applied to health belief systems to give more or less credence to them. For example, claiming to be rationalistic implies being logical and scientific, having evidence of cause and effect, being testable and proven; whilst mystical suggests magic, witchcraft and being metaphysical, unproven and unscientific. Furthermore, we can note a value judgement being applied to medical approaches that claim to be reductionist (we understand the component parts) and holistic (we do not understand how the parts affect the whole). Consider Vignette 4.4 which provides an example of how two approaches can be successfully combined.

Vignette 4.4

Mariyah, a 14-year-old Indian girl living with her parents who emigrated to the UK four years ago, is admitted to the Intensive Care Unit in a serious state of septicaemia. Following tests and 48 hours of intravenous antibiotics, she is deteriorating and grave concerns for her life are expressed by the doctor. The family contact the local Shaman who arrives that evening with a small bottle containing a clear fluid. He informs everyone that the potion contains a secret ingredient that will cure Mariyah and wishes to give her a few drops immediately before she dies. The medical staff ask what the potion contains but the Sharman refuses to tell them, claiming that its secret is its potency and once revealed it will no longer be effective. The family agree but the medical staff do not. The Consultant is called and suggests that the potion be analysed in the laboratory. The Shaman refuses to hand the potion over and outlines the urgency of administering it to Mariyah. The medical staff are worried that the potion will harm Mariyah but as it is only a few drops they relent and agree once a disclaimer form is signed. The potion is given to Mariyah and by the following morning an improvement in her condition is noted. Prior to being discharged, a case conference is called during which the medical staff state that Mariyah was cured by the antibiotics and life support; the Shaman states that she was cured, as expected, by the secret potion and the smiling parents state that they were pleased that Mariyah was going home.

Conclusion

In this chapter, we note the interplay of numerous aspects that work together to form an understanding of what it means to be human in relation to states of health and illness. We choose to view ourselves and others either in reductionist terms or in a holistic manner, or sometimes in a combination of both. In any event, health and social care decisions are based on the underpinning values that govern our culture, with its beliefs, traditions and norms. Our belief in science tends towards an explanation of illness and social difficulty based on the logic of cause and effect. However, values we espouse in terms of the value of the individual urge us ever closer to a values-based approach to care.

References

Aristotle (1998) *The Metaphysics*. Harmondsworth: Penguin.

Bach, S., Kessler, I. and Heron, P. (2008) 'Role redesign in a modernised NHS: the case of health care assistants', *Human Resource Management Journal*, 18(2): 171–87.

Bakker, I. and Miller, R. (1996) 'Escape from Fordism', in R. Boyer and D. Drache (eds) *States Against Market*. London: Routledge, pp. 334–56.

Bauman, Z. (1996) *Modernity and the Holocaust*. Oxford: Blackwell.

Beauchamp, T. and Childress, J. (1994) *Principles of Biomedical Ethics*, 4th edition. Oxford: Oxford University Press.

Blass, T. (2002) 'The man who shocked the world', *Psychology Today*, 35(2): 68.

Blickstein, I. (2007) 'Litigation in multiple pregnancy and birth', *Clinics in Perinatology*, 34(2): 319–27.

Bolton, S.C. (2003) 'Multiple roles? Nurses as managers in the NHS', *International Journal of Public Sector Management*, 16(2): 122–30.

Buber, M. (1937) *I and Thou*. Edinburgh: T. and T. Clark.

Calne, S. (1994) 'Dehumanisation in intensive care', *Nursing Times*, 90(17): 31–3.

Carvel, J. (2008) 'Nurses to be rated on how compassionate and smiley they are', *The Guardian*, 18 June. Available at: http://www.guardian.co.uk/society/2008/jun/18/nhs60.nhs1 [accessed 6 March 2010]

Clark, D. (2002) 'Between hope and acceptance: the medicalisation of dying', *British Medical Journal*, 324(7342): 905–7.

Cooper, M.C. (1993) 'The intersection of technology and care in the ICU', *Advances in Nursing Science*, 15(3): 23–32.

Cooper, R., Griffith, C., Malik, R., Obee, P. and Looker, N. (2003) 'Monitoring the effectiveness of cleaning in four British hospitals', *American Journal of Infection Control,* 35(5): 338–41.

Corrigan, I., Samuelson, K.A., Fridlund, B. and Thome, B. (2007) 'The meaning of posttraumatic stress-reactions following critical illness or injury and intensive care treatment', *Intensive Care Nursing,* 23(4): 206–15.

Cowan, J. and Anthony, S. (2008) 'Problems with complaint handling: expectations and outcomes', *Clinical Governance: An International Journal,* 13(2): 164–8.

Culbertson, L. (2007) 'Human-ness, "dehumanisation" and performance enhancement', *Sport, Ethics and Philosophy,* 1(2): 195–217.

Fendrick, A.M., Smith, D.G., Chernow, M.E. and Shah, S.N. (2001) 'A benefit-based co-pay for prescription drugs: patient contribution based on total benefits, not drug acquisition cost', *American Journal of Management Care,* 7: 861–7.

Finster, M. and Wood, M. (2005) 'The APGAR score has survived the test of time: classic papers revisited', *Anesthesiology,* 102(4): 855–7.

Fisher, M. (2006) *Beating Anger: The Eight Point Plan for Coping with Rage.* New York: Random House.

Foucault, M. (1973) *The Birth of the Clinic: An Archaeology of Medical Perception.* New York: Pantheon.

Floyd, T. (2008) 'Medical malpractice: trends in litigation', *Gastroenterology,* 134(7): 1822–5.

Giddens, A. (1997) *Sociology,* 2nd edition. Cambridge: Polity Press.

Giddens, A. (2000) *Sociology,* 3rd edition. Cambridge: Polity Press.

Greenstein, A., Bym, J., Zhang, L., Swedish, K., Jahn, A. and Divino, C. (2003) 'Risk factors for the development of fulminant Clostridium difficile colitis', *Surgery,* 143(5): 623–9.

Haney, C., Banks, C. and Zimbardo, P.G. (1973) 'Interpersonal dynamics in a simulated prison', paper presented at Stanford University. National Criminal Justice Reference Service No. 010301.

Hart, G. and Wellings, K. (2002) 'Sexual behaviour and its medicalisation: in sickness and in health', *British Medical Journal,* 324(7342): 896–900.

Hawking, S.W. (1995) *A Brief History of Time: From the Big Bang to Black Holes.* New York: Random House.

Heath, C., Luff, P. and Svenson, M.S. (2003) 'Technology and medical practice', *Sociology of Health and Illness,* 25(3): 75–96.

Hemachandra, A.H., Howards, P.P., Furth, S.L. and Klebanoff, M.A. (2007) 'Birth weight, postnatal growth and risk for high blood pressure at 7 years of age: results from the Collaborative Perinatal Project', *Pediatrics,* 119(6): 1264–70.

Herrick, J. (2005) *Humanism: An Introduction*. London: Routledge.

Holden, R.J. (2007) 'Responsibility and autonomous nursing practice', *Journal of Advanced Nursing*, 16(4): 398–403.

Hutchinson, D.S. (1997) *Plato: Complete Works*. Indianapolis, IN: Hackett Publishing Co.

Ideker, T. and Sharan, R. (2008) 'Protein networks in disease', *Genome Research*, 18(4): 644–52.

Illich, I. (1976) *Limits to Medicine – Medical Nemesis: The Expropriation of Health*. London: Marion Boyers.

James, S. (1984) *The Content of Social Explanation*. Cambridge: Cambridge University Press.

Keen, A. (2006) A qualitative exploration of the concept of dehumanisation as experienced by nurses within the context of information systems. Unpublished Master of Science thesis, Faculty of Health and Social Care, University of Chester.

Kurtz, P. (2006) *What is Secular Humanism?* New York: Prometheus.

Lemos, R.M. (1995) *The Nature of Value: Axiological Investigations*. Cambridge: Cambridge University Press.

Likhterman, L.B. (2005) 'Human face of neurosurgery: possibilities and problems', *Acta Neurochirugica*, 124(2–4): 179–81.

Lundy, M.C. (2007) 'Nursing beyond Fordism', *Employee Responsibilities and Rights Journal*, 9(2): 163–71.

Lyotard, J.-F. (1990) *Heidegger and 'the Jews'*. Minneapolis: University of Minneapolis Press.

Maiese, M. (2003) 'Dehumanization', *Beyond Intractability*. Available at: www. beyondintractability.org/essay/dehumanization/?nid=1082 [accessed 1 December 2009]

Manser, T. and Staender, S. (2005) 'Aftermath of an adverse event: supporting health care professionals to meet patient expectations through open disclosure', *Acta Anaesthesiologica Scandinavica*, 49(6): 728–34.

Mason, T. and Whitehead, E. (2003) *Thinking Nursing*. Maidenhead: Open University Press.

McPhail, K. (1999) *The Other Objective of Ethics Education: Rehumanising the Accounting Profession*. Glasgow: University of Glasgow Press.

ME Association (2009) *About ME*. Available at: www.meassociation.org.uk/ content/blogcategory/38/173/ [accessed 1 December 2009]

Menon, S. (2006) 'Do reality TV shows dehumanise?', *The Economic Times,* 23rd August Available at: http://economictimes.indiatimes.com/ articleshow/1917286.cms [accessed 1 December 2009]

Milgram, S. (1974) *Obedience to Authority*. London: Harper Row.

Nachmias, C. and Nachmias, D. (1981) *Research Methods in the Social Sciences.* London: Edward Arnold.

Norman, R. (2004) *On Humanism (Thinking in Action).* New York: Prometheus.

Parsons, T.S. (1951) *The Social System.* Glencoe, IL: Free Press.

Pearcey, P. (2007) 'Tasks and routines in 21st century nursing: student nurses' perceptions', *British Journal of Nursing,* 16(5): 296–300.

Pearcey, P. (2008) 'Shifting roles in nursing: does role extension require role abdication', *Journal of Clinical Nursing,* 17(10): 1320–6.

Pilgrim, D. and Bentall, R. (1999) 'The medicalisation of misery: a critical realist analysis of the concept of depression', *Journal of Mental Health,* 8(3): 261–74.

Purtilo, R. (1993) *Ethical Dimensions in the Health Professions,* 2nd edition. Phildelphia, PA: W.B. Saunders.

Rajmil, L., Herdman, M., Fernandez de Sanmamed, M., Detmar, S., Bruil, J., Ravens-Sieberer, U., Bullinger, M., Simeoni, M. and Auquier, P. (2004) 'Generic health-related quality of life instruments in children and adolescents: a qualitative analysis of content', *Journal of Adolescent Health,* 34(1): 37–45.

Richman, J. (1987) *Medicine and Health.* London: Longman.

Rosenberg, A. (2006) *Darwinian Reductionism or How to Stop Worrying and Love Molecular Biology.* Chicago, IL: University of Chicago Press.

Rowson, R.H. (1990) *An Intoduction to Ethics for Nurses.* Harrow: Scutari Press.

Schwartz, S.H. (1992) 'Universals in the content and structure of values: theoretical advances and empirical tests in 20 countries', in M. Zana (ed.) *Advances in Experimental Social Psychology.* San Diego, CA: Academic Press, pp. 1–62.

Schwartz, S.H. (1994) 'Beyond individualism/collectivism: new dimensions of values', in U. Kim, H.C. Triandis, C. Kagitcibasi, S.C. Choi and G. Yoon (eds) *Individualism and Collectivism: Theory Application and Methods.* Newbury Park, CA: Sage, pp. 85–122.

Schwartz, S.H., Roccas, S., Lilach, S. and Knafo, A. (2002) 'The big five personality factors and personal values', *Personality and Social Psychology Bulletin,* 28(6): 789–801.

Shaw, P. and Mountain, D. (2007) 'The medical model is dead – long live the medical model', *The British Journal of Psychiatry,* 191: 375–7.

Shaw, B., Cheater, F., Baker, R., Gillies, C., Hearnshaw, H., Flottorp, S. and Roberson, N. (2008) 'Tailored interventions to overcome identified barriers to change: effects on professional practice and health care outcomes',

Cochrane Database of Systematic Reviews, Issue 3. Chichester: John Wiley and Sons.

Smith, R. (1997) 'The future of healthcare systems', *British Medical Journal,* 314: 1495.

Szasz, T. (1974) *Ideology and Insanity: Essays on the Psychiatric Dehumanisation of Man.* London: Marion Boyars.

Tschudin, V. and Marks-Maran, D. (1993) *Ethics: A Primer for Nurses.* London: Ballière Tindall.

Warne, T. and McAndrew, S. (2008) 'Value', in E. Whitehead-Mason, A. McIntosh, A. Bryan and T. Mason (eds) *Key Concepts in Nursing*, London: Sage, pp. 315–21.

Williamson, A. and Hoggart, B. (2005) 'Pain: a review of three commonly used pain rating scales', *Journal of Clinical Nursing*, 14(7): 798–804.

Wirth, A. (2007) 'Victor E. Frankl and "The Responsible Self"', *Educational Theory*, 12(4): 241–6.

Zimbardo, P.G., Maslach, C. and Haney, C. (1999) 'Reflections on the Stanford Prison Experiment', in T. Blass (ed.) *Obedience to Authority: Current Perspectives on the Milgram Paradigm.* Mahwah, NJ: Lawrence Erlbaum, pp. 193–238.

5 Valuing Professional Judgement

Jill McCarthy, Pauline Alexander, Moyra Baldwin and Jan Woodhouse

Professional practice in the caring professions involves applying knowledge and skills to effect service users' health, wellness and well-being. A cornerstone of clinical professional practice is expertise: the means by which individual practitioners make decisions, based on their professional judgement. Professional practitioners in health and social care exercise both independence and interdependence in their professional activities underpinned by their professional values, knowledge and confidence. The pressures of corporate managerial control and external influences such as the evidence-based practice movement impinge on, and constrain, professional practice. The nature of professional practice is that it requires professional expertise, clinical judgement and decision making. Values-based care in respect of professional judgement is explored by examining the nature of professional practice and professionalism, the application of professional judgement, intuition, and mentorship and patronage. Professional judgement is the foundation of values-based care and this chapter, through highlighting the importance of this judgement, reinforces the need for this new health care policy.

Professional Practice

Professional practice and professionalism have over decades been defined in terms of traits, status, power or control. Elements of professional practice include mission, mastery, orientation towards problem solving, and critical as well as creative application of knowledge. These elements are acquired following lengthy formal training and continued self-enhancement (Fish and Coles, 1998; Houle, cited by Leddy and Pepper, 1993; see also Health Professions Council; Nursing and Midwifery Council; General Medical Council and General Social Care Council) and are further supported by systems of governance that accredit and certify practitioners as competent. Thus, professionals' work is distinguished from that of others, and standards are secured and reinforced by means of legal systems that penalise the incompetent and unethical practitioner. It is evident that the public acknowledges professionals as knowledgeable practitioners, sanctioned to apply their professional judgement and to exercise professional autonomy in the pursuit of excellence. The professional is therefore afforded trust and confidence, and this was indeed the case until the latter half of the 20th century. Public trust, of late, has been eroded and professionals find themselves under siege, according to Fish and Coles (1998), which is good reason to examine the nature of professional practice, expose the underpinning beliefs associated with it in the caring professions and articulate the inherent values. At the heart of professional practice, however, lies the primacy of the service users' best interests.

As we have seen in earlier chapters, for too long there has been increasing criticism of the professions and professional practice by a strengthening consumerist movement, resulting in an erosion of professional independence and autonomy. Criticism, it appears, that has been founded on the perception that professionals have behaved out of self-interest, rather than altruism, that has disempowered the service user. Yet it is the very same consumerism and marketplace philosophy that undermines professional practice. Professionals, before the rise of evidence-based practice, practised according to the available evidence and expert opinion, in order to provide service users with effective treatments and interventions. The evidence was founded on personal expertise and knowledge, gained through experience with service users and through discussions with professional colleagues. Professional practice involves interdependence as well as independence and enables practitioners to develop confidence in their professional ability whilst also retaining the confidence of the service user, and peers. Such is the nature of professional practice that it mirrors current inter-professional working and learning which is expected of practitioners in the caring professions in contemporary society, and is essential to individual service users' health, wellness and well-being, as well as that of society.

Programmes of education provide professionals with a knowledge base for practice. This knowledge facilitates confidence, competence and the development of expertise. According to Glazer (cited by Schön, 1991: 23), a profession's knowledge base has four essential characteristics: specialised, bounded, scientific and standardised. Contrary to the connotation of unsophisticated acceptance and application of guidelines so often required of contemporary evidence-based health and social care practice, the standardised knowledge noted by Glazer (cited by Schön, 1991) is neither static nor, indeed, standard. It is about recognising that many health and social care problems share similar aspects, such that the professional practitioner is able to apply principles to practice in order to offer appropriate interventions or solutions to problems. Thus, the professional practitioner practising in the caring professions not only demonstrates expertise, but also excellence by being flexible in the application of acquired professional knowledge. Mastery is displayed by the use of basic and applied science theory: key elements of professional knowledge. The nature of professional practice and, by inference, the value of professional judgement, thus requires the exercise of higher-order cognitive skills. It involves knowing HOW and WHEN to use the knowledge whereby the professional practitioner demonstrates discriminant use of knowledge in enabling individualised, personalised, high-quality health and social care. This is a partnership, combining the service user's knowledge, decision making, problem solving, judgement, confidence and expertise with that of the professional practitioner.

Professional practice, however, is not merely about the practitioner ingesting vast amounts of knowledge. Of significance to professional practice is the ability to recognise the difference between relevant and irrelevant material in order that the practitioner can act with timeliness and propriety. The professional practitioner is knowledgeable, able to integrate salient aspects from a range of sources, and applies judgement to problem solving both critically and creatively. It is the reason why professional practitioners need to undertake a lengthy period of training. Unlike vocational training where someone performs skills to perfection, professional training incorporates education such that the professional practitioner not only learns skills but also knowledge, and by this we could say the wisdom to know WHEN and HOW to do something and, perhaps as importantly, when NOT to. This is the reason why, as yet, it has not been possible to build a practically intelligent robot. In the field of Artificial Intelligence, there is the concept of the Philosopher's Frame, and Dennett's (2005) story about the frame problem illustrates the point well (see Dennett, 2005 for a fuller explanation). R_1, the first robot, failed to recognise that its action would cause self-destruction. The next robot, R_1D_1, would deduce the implications of its actions before acting, but deliberating for too long on irrelevance also caused its destruction. Robot R_2D_1 (robot-relevant-deducer) was programmed not only to recognise the relevant and irrelevant implications of its actions but also to ignore the latter. Whilst working hard, sifting through the thousands of irrelevant consequences so that it could place each on its list of those it needed to ignore, it too came to the same sad demise and was destroyed.

Professional practice operates within an environment that is dynamic. It is not context-free and herein lies the point. Irrelevances are excluded, but how a professional achieves the ability to ignore the irrelevant aspects in a given experience with a service user is complex. If, as we have asserted above, professional practitioners exercise the discriminant and creative application of knowledge, then professional practice values include the concepts of professional judgement and individuality. Long before evidence-based practice was pedalled as essential to National Health Service and Social Service care, Elstein and Bordage (cited by Harbison, 1991) explored expert physicians' judgement. Based on their professional knowledge and experience, these experts believed they were intuitive in their decision making, yet analysis revealed that they used a hypothetico-deductive approach to clinical decisions. Early in their meetings with service users, using basic and applied science knowledge, they made a number of hypotheses which then guided their practice. They sought out further cues that would allow them to either support or reject each hypothesis. Using the skills associated with higher-order cognitive thinking, practitioners analysed problems and by their discretionary use of knowledge, appraised and evaluated their findings to give both direction and eventual conclusion to effecting quality health and social care. When knowledge is used discriminantly, the professional requires both the confidence and the freedom to exercise it. Herein lies autonomy, but also the value of professional integrity which is one of the many crucial ingredients of professional practice. The failure of integrity in an accredited professional destroys public trust and perhaps it is understandable that a degree of scepticism is the result, and thus a resort to evidence-based practice.

Sources of knowledge are manifold and the evidence-based practice movement has advanced as essential that knowledge be gained by means of research. For example, see Sackett et al. (1997) who espouse attentive, explicit and discerning application of best evidence to the care of service users. This appeal to evidence-based practice paradoxically militates against individual professional autonomy and integrity as it demands that professionals apply research-based evidence on the one hand yet requires critical and judicious scrutiny of the evidence on the other. This should imply that professionals can exercise their autonomy by rejecting as well as accepting aspects of evidence. Yet this is often not the case in practice, as witnessed by the protocols and procedures advanced by National Health Service Trusts, Social Services departments and government directives in the form of National Service Frameworks, Care Pathways and Single Assessment Processes. Buetow and Kenealy (2000) remind us that evidence is obtained from both scientific and non-scientific sources of knowledge, thus professional practitioners need to base their decisions on their independent and autonomous judgement: the application of science and the 'technical rationality' (Schön 1991) that professionals practice when engaged in problem solving. But it is more than this, as noted by Luntley (2007) – it is experiential knowledge.

Professional practice is complex, involving actions that are geared to developing and sustaining rapport between the professional and service user, to enable therapeutic relationships and interactions in which there is mutual respect. It is by its nature subjective and value-laden (Dowie cited by Colyer and Kamath, 1999), demanding sensitive application of personal, professional practice knowledge. Experiential knowledge is thus the crux of professional practice. Practice problems cannot be solved by single, disconnected solutions chosen from a range of options rather like choosing a recipe from a cookbook, or the robot actions noted previously. It is misguided to believe that the value-free knowledge gained from evidence-based practice, audit or related data can be applied to problems in order to reduce risks and prevent errors or care that fall short of excellent. Practice in caring professions requires appreciation of the subjective nature of human interactions and the judicious application of knowledge to affect therapeutic relationships. It is about professional clinical expertise, the application and use of experiential and expert knowledge, and the freedom to exercise professional judgement with each unique interaction.

Inherent in this complex interaction is the recognition that the professional and service user are both experts: expert in their own domain, with mutual confidence in each other's desire to develop a healthy partnership. Whilst Savage (1993: 6) explored the philosophical assumptions of various nurse–service user relationship models, the assertions about caring equally apply to any health or social care discipline – it 'has nothing to do with possessing privileged information that increases one's control and domination of another. Rather expert caring ... unleashes the possibilities inherent in the self and the situation'.

Vignette 5.1 illustrates health and social care professionals using their skill and judgement to ensure the best outcome for the individual service. This is an example of values-based care whereby professionals marry their values with those of the service user to obtain the optimum outcome for that particular individual.

Vignette 5.1

I was diagnosed with breast cancer five years ago and have developed bone secondaries causing pain in my back and legs. I take the regular medication prescribed and can walk with a mobility aid. At a ward round, the doctor, nurse and physiotherapist told me they had discussed my care-plan at their multidisciplinary team meeting.

(Continued)

(Continued)

One of the choices regarding my care included staying in bed and not walking (weight-bearing) anymore, because my bones are 'fragile' and this was presented as the safest option. The team however values me as an individual and appreciates that I need symptom relief that allows me as much normality as possible in my day-to-day life, even if this is not in line with the best available evidence. With the team's support I am to continue mobilising as before.

If the professionals were to uncritically apply basic biological science, due to the strong risk of fractured pelvis, then I would have been confined to bed-rest which would have left me feeling alienated and upset. Knowing HOW and WHEN to use knowledge the team informed me of the facts, enabled me to make the choice and plan care in accordance with my personality and my situation. Influences on presenting bed-rest as the best evidence-based intervention could be due to rationing services and, more likely, the potential for litigation that another person in similar circumstances might consider. The professionals practised according to their value system which involved evaluating the importance of trust in the service user-practitioner relationship, discretion, risk analysis and confident expert judgement.

Expertise and Experience in Professional Judgement

Clinical expertise is developed through experience and can only be successfully applied by the professional using past knowledge and practical skills creatively and flexibly to new or novel situations. The professional becomes expert by virtue of the number of previous opportunities whereby they have applied knowledge and skills to achieve successful outcomes. However, this is not to suggest that expertise is developed through repetition alone, but more specifically that the application of judgement, which embraces both conscious and unconscious thought processes and includes holistic assessment, may be brought into play in each situation.

Gadamer (cited by Melnyk and Fineout-Overholt, 2005: 170) expresses the view that:

> Experience is never a mere passage of time or exposure to an event. To qualify as experience it requires a turning around of preconceptions, expectations, sets and routines or adding some new insights to a particular practical situation.

Experiential learning is at the heart of improving clinical judgement and it is the ability to harness previous knowledge and experience in a discerning, thoughtful manner that can enable the practitioner to develop expertise. The concept of reflective practice has a pivotal place in enabling practitioners to make sense of their practice. Schön's (1983, 1987) concepts of both reflection-in-action (thinking creatively whilst carrying out an action) and reflection-on-action (thinking back on actions taken) serve as means to enable the practitioner to continually modify their actions as expertise evolves.

Using reflection-in-action allows the practitioner to develop the ability to make rapid judgements and decisions in problematic situations and through this some degree of expertise is gained. Benner's (1984) work on the development of expert practice sees expertise emerging from the ability not only to apply technical knowledge, but also the ability to understand each situation through the assimilation of a wide range of experience and using this to assign specific meaning. Benner et al. (1996: 2) dispute that clinical decision making arises out of 'the rational selection of alternatives from a set of mutually exclusive possibilities', but rather that this focus on conscious analysis ignores the non-conscious, non-analytical aspects of judgement that form expert function.

Dunne (cited by Melnyk and Fineout-Overholt, 2005) outlines the distinction espoused by Aristotle between the 'techne' which involves the art or skill applied and the 'phronesis' which is the professional judgement applied to clinical practice. Dowie and Macnaughton (2000) view good clinical judgement as being evidence-based with a fusion between technical judgement and humane judgement and also the application of ethical sensitivity. Rational scientific knowledge and research encompassed within evidence-based practice can support practitioners in their decision making, however this has limitations and cannot be totally value-free, therefore it can be restrictive in enabling the practitioner to respond to every facet of their clinical practice.

Practitioners who wish to embed a sound evidence base within their practice will find it difficult unless they address the clear need to consider the corresponding values-based practice which complements the growing body of evidence in decision making. Petrova et al. (2006) suggest that values-based practice is a valuable support to clinical decision making where complex and conflicting values arise. Each professional encounter with service users in health and social care settings is a unique situation which requires the professional to draw upon a vast range of knowledge and experience. The uniqueness of each encounter may be compared with the infinite varieties of patterns seen in a microscopic view of snowflakes.

Health is a highly disputed concept which can have a range of interpretations and definitions applied to it. Exploration of the concept reveals perceptions that extend from the view that health equates with an absence of disease, to the functional view that it is an ability to cope with daily activity, or that health is about positive wellness and spirituality. It is not surprising that given this array of interpretations of health, there are many views as to how this can be best achieved. It is essential to recognise that within the clinical encounter, service users, carers and practitioners will all have their own perceptions, values and preferences. It is imperative that due consideration is given to such concerns to enable the construction of a shared view which can assist in the achievement of a successful outcome.

It is suggested by Woodbridge and Fulford (2004) that there are key prerequisites to implementing a values-based practice approach, the most important of these being the need to consider the service user's values as the first priority. This can only be achieved through the use of good communication and establishing a rapport with those concerned in order to enable an effective dialogue to take place. In order to fully engage with service users, use professional judgement and apply clinical decision making appropriately using problem-solving skills, there is a need for an atmosphere of openness and transparency.

Acknowledgement of the wide range of diversity, and valuing this in order to work in such a way as to eradicate inequality, discrimination and stigma, will enhance equitable access to health and social care and enable the development of services which are truly responsive to service users' needs. Professionals will need to acknowledge not only the personal values that they themselves hold, but more importantly those held by service users and their families and carers. These diverse perspectives also need to be balanced with the perspectives of other professionals within the multi-disciplinary team who may be involved in the care of the service user. Partnership working between all parties which is based on respect, trust and a willingness to work constructively to overcome tensions which may arise as a result of differences in values, perspectives or expectations, is vital for the successful achievement of positive outcomes. Health and social care professionals have both a shared and unique culture with specific values which will be shaped by legal, ethical and professional codes of practice. The professional will need to be constantly aware and mindful of their individual accountability in decision making and how this is influenced by their personal values. Within multi-disciplinary teams, there needs to be acknowledgement of power differentials and every attempt must be made to address these concerns to enable each party to contribute fully to the service user's benefit.

Contemporary health and social care policy encompasses the ideal of service user choice and as scientific knowledge expands, there is the potential to create new options and choices. This may be choice in terms of time, place or duration of care and could also involve choice around which professional the service user wishes to consult and the type of service delivery. Health and social care professionals have an important role to play in facilitating access to high-quality care and in ensuring that the services offered provide evidence-based care which also takes account of individual service users' needs. The goals set by service users may or may not be compatible with those of the professional; this may arise either because they have unrealistic expectations of the services or because professionals fail to articulate their goals, and allow their knowledge of resource implications to constrain their practice. There is a fine balance to be achieved between the empowerment process which enables individuals to play an active role in decision making and the identifiable risk which may readily exist when their decisions do not adhere to evidence-based conformity. It is essential that the notion of one-size-fits-all solutions or, only one possible interpretation of how a rational clinical decision is reached, is challenged in order to maintain the freedom to make decisions and negotiate these decisions, in a service user's best interests. This process may require the practitioner to initially abandon any preconceived ideas and values from their past experience, in order to be amenable to all potential directions and to be able to give the service user's view priority.

Evidence-based guidelines have a place in the decision-making process and can support the practitioner, whilst ensuring that there is adherence to protocol in terms of acceptable standards of care and clinical governance. The strength of research-based evidence to support guidelines can provide the practitioner with a degree of confidence in their decision making, allowing them to justify their decisions and actions within their professional practice norms. It is for this reason that the use of evidence-based guidelines has been adopted as a mechanism to spread good health and social care practice and to disseminate research.

The use of evidence-based guidelines to practically support decision making has been evident within the field of remote assessment, where computer decision support software has been developed to assist practitioners in assessment. Whilst such tools can be valuable in providing a standardised response, they cannot have the sensitivity to incorporate individual values into the decision-making equation. Pearson et al. (2007) describe how the use of clinical decision support systems in health care can facilitate decision making and induce change in intervention or process-based behaviour, but they caution that there are limitations in assessment or diagnostic activities. It is important that there is an acknowledgement of both the limitations and the benefits of using adjuncts to clinical decision making in the form of clinical decision support software. The use of this tool in the hands of inexperienced practitioners could prove to be detrimental to safe decision making if the ability to override the protocols in the light of knowledge and experience is not exercised appropriately.

Vignette 5.2 assists in highlighting how complex clinical decision making can prove to be.

Vignette 5.2

I guess I hadn't really taken in the enormity of what was happening. Bobby at 16 is my youngest child, he was always a sensitive boy, he seems to tune into my moods. When I divorced Pete, Bobby was distraught and seemed to shut off to me. His diagnosis of Non Hodgkin's Lymphoma was a huge shock; I hadn't had time to take it all in before his treatment started. Bobby shrugged his shoulders and dismissed my fussing over him, appearing resigned to it all. The first dose of chemotherapy hit him like a sledgehammer; despite the anti-sickness drugs he vomited incessantly, he was a dreadful colour. I convinced myself he was dying.

When I rang through to the out-of-hours service, the process of getting through frustrated me and by the time I reached the nurse I was hysterical and extremely rude. The questions were endless; I understand that they need to ask, but all I wanted was for Bobby's vomiting to be dealt with. Thankfully, they came out to the house eventually to give him an injection, but it took a while to take effect.

This story highlights several crucial elements, not least the tensions between a teenage boy striving for independence and acceptance of his illness and his mother's understandable anxiety. The mother, in a nurturing capacity, wants to advocate on her son's behalf in order to address the distressing side effects of the chemotherapy. There is a clear need for recognition that both the service user and his mother require information to enable them to understand the diagnosis, prognosis and treatment of the illness. In addition to this are the concerns of the nurse working in a remote assessment situation using decision support software which promotes evidence-based guidelines which can, and should be, overridden in the context of the presenting case. This complex case concerning individual problems cannot easily be solved using algorithms based on presenting symptoms, despite the fact that sound evidence-based rationales underpin the suggested advice and outcome. It is in such a situation that the practitioner will need to draw upon all previous knowledge skills and experience to enable the most acceptable outcome to be reached. It is through the ability to view this situation in its entirety, with focus on communication, information gathering, problem solving and timely intervention, that the service users' needs can be met.

It can be seen, therefore, that values-based care takes us beyond evidence-based practice. A balance needs to be struck between the two in order that decisions are reached using each practitioner's experience and expertise to fully enhance the service user's health or social care encounter. Service users need to be given the freedom to exercise autonomy in deciding how their needs are best met; equally, health and social care professionals need to have a degree of freedom to exercise professional autonomy in negotiating the best outcomes for their service users.

Intuition in Professional Judgement

Within the writings on professional judgement, the notion of intuition is often explored. This section will consider the definitions of intuition, iden-tify the cognitive processes of intuition and consider issues of its application to practice.

A colleague, who teaches research and evidence-based practice, discusses intuition at the start of a module on the topic of evidence-based practice. The students are asked to debate the question: 'Is intuition as valid as evidence-based practice?' and to come up with reasons for their answers. A lively debate usually ensues as argument and counter-argument are given. At the end of the debate, the class is given a free vote and the teacher records the votes. It is reported that the novice student nurses overwhelmingly come down in favour of intuition being as valid as evidence-based practice, although they always add the rider that judgements in practice are probably a combination of the two. However, when the same exercise was carried out with registered nurses, the opposite was found, that is, they considered that evidence-based practice was more valid than intuitive practice.

Just what would account for this shift in attitude from the novice nurse to that of the experienced practitioner? In order to explore this, a definition of intuition must be sought. Benner and Tanner (1987) were early writers on the use of intuition in nursing, and their definition, that intuition is 'understanding without rationale', is often quoted in subsequent texts (Banning, 2007; Effken, 2001; Perry, 2000). However, Effken (2001), following an extensive literature search, noted that there were at least 23 definitions of intuition, covering a span of 40+ years. These date from Polayni's 1958 version of tacit knowledge, through several 1980s theorists (including Benner and Tanner, 1987) to a definition that intuition is predicated in sound knowledge and reasoning (as suggested by Schrader and Fisher); and on into the 1990s with Rew defining it as an innate knowledge and Meerabeau calling it artistry (all cited by Effken, 2001). Cioffi (1997) adds to the definitions, and notes that intuitive judgements lack underlying conscious processes and are not, therefore, explicable in a tangible manner.

The search for an all-encompassing definition continues into the 21st century, with refinements of the concept being recorded by Hansten and Washburn in 2000 (cited by Effken, 2001) as an ability to discern and noting that it comes with a gut feeling. Callaghan (2007) expands on a definition, by giving a list of characteristics that try to sum up the notion of intuition, including: whim, habit, extrasensory perception, telepathy, mysticism and female intuition. It is important to note here the reference to gender made within these characteristics. This issue is explored below.

From these readings, it can be seen that defining intuition has been a focus of academics for many years and that the debate still rages. Researchers, building on the knowledge base of their predecessors, have more of an understanding of this ethereal concept and have attempted to break it down, describe it and measure its use in practice.

Aspects of intuition

The early work of Benner and Tanner (1987) discusses six key aspects of intuitive judgement in their analysis of intuition in nursing:

1. *Pattern recognition*, they suggest, comes from repeated exposure to an experience – noticing that there may be subtle differences between those experiences which would not be evident in a textbook case.
2. *Similarity recognition* is where the practitioner is reminded of similar service users who had problems. This capacity to recall similar episodes also helps to note *dissimilar* situations. Both help to open up lines of enquiry (formulating a hypothesis).
3. *Commonsense understanding* is where the practitioner uses *all* the information about the service user to come to a decision, rather than relying on reductionist information, such as bio-physical test results. Using intuitive practice, the practitioner will draw on knowledge of the bio-psycho-social-spiritual aspects of an individual service user to gain an understanding of their current status.
4. *Skilled know-how* is where the intuitive practitioner knows how the body's systems work and can envisage what the service user is experiencing, for example if a nurse is passing a catheter, s/he can visualise the hidden

structures that the catheter is in touch with, knows when it is inserted to the right degree and, therefore, when the retaining balloon is inflated, knows that it is sitting in the right position. Nurses who have this notion of embodiment will physically wince if they are told the tale of the service user who had their catheter withdrawn without deflating the balloon first.

5. *Sense of salience* is an understanding that some aspects of a service user's condition are more important than others. It goes beyond checklist practice, where service users are assessed using criteria. A sense of salience will draw on other information rather than sticking to the criteria.

6. *Deliberate rationality* is a strategy to adopt where there is a risk of 'tunnel thinking' – would the interpretation of the situation change if a different perspective is taken? Formulating different hypotheses is part of this process – what if it is this, what if it is that? This supports the case for discussion with a colleague, perhaps from a different discipline, to aid hypothesis formation.

Benner and Tanner (1987) question whether intuition can be taught. They note that attention should be paid to teaching methods, with developing an inquiring mind being more important than promoting a 'checklist mentality'. They argue that the use of case studies, feedback, preceptoring and validation by expert practitioners, helps in the processes of enquiry and pattern recognition skills. They conclude that 'intuitive knowledge and analytical reasoning are *not* in either/or opposition; they can and often do work together' (Benner and Tanner, 1987: 31). Cioffi (1997) further explores the concept of intuition and reports on two types of intuition found in the literature: cognitive inference and Gestalt intuition.

- *Cognitive inference* is the rapid assimilation of visual and verbal cues, which may be at a subliminal level. These are then forgotten when consciously considering the decision-making process.
- *Gestalt intuition* is where 'gaps, missing pieces or hidden relationships are detected' from a plethora of information that then emerges as a pattern.

More recently, and still on the elusive track of defining intuition, Banning (2007) researched the decision-making process in nurses. Here she discusses the:

- *Information-process model*, which, Banning claims, is rooted in medical decision making. The individual thinks through a number of decision trees in order to arrive at a final outcome, for example, 'If I do ... then what will be the outcome?'
- Alongside the information-process model is the *analytical, decision-making model*. The underpinning aspect of this model is that a rationality of thought can be followed to the point of the decision. Repeatedly asking the question 'Why ... ?' may help in establishing whether this model has been used.

- Both of the above consider the *hypothetico-deductive approach,* which requires:
  - Cue recognition or acquisition: what do you see?
  - Hypothesis generation: what could be the reason for what you see?
  - Cue interpretation: does the reason match up with what you see?
  - Hypothesis evaluation: depending on whether the cues confirm (reason does match) or reject (reason doesn't match) the initial hypothesis.

Banning (2007) reports that nurses may struggle, when decision making, to generate a hypothesis and that using decision trees (*does x exist – yes or no?*) helps to formulate a diagnosis. She notes that qualified nurses, when administering medication, used the above approach, as opposed to using intuitive practices. Intuitive practices, Banning states, are decision-making when the cues are rapidly changing or textbook cues are deemed inappropriate combined with a lack of hypothesis testing. Here, the nurse reverts to Benner and Tanner's (1987) definition of 'understanding without rationale' and considers the service user with immediacy and holistically rather than with linear, analytical reasoning (Rew cited by Banning, 2007).

Applying intuitive practice

Cioffi (1997) records that intuitive practice or judgement was, in the past, associated with gender (the notion of female intuition) and that it existed in parallel with the male-dominated scientific world. Science, after all, seeks to provide answers to hypotheses; it is objective and logical. If females still arrived at the same answers as their male counterparts in the absence of scientific methods and logic, this suggested a mystery and we see the terms 'mysticism', 'extra sensory perception (ESP)' or 'female intuition' being applied to the phenomenon. Rashotte and Carnevale (2004) propose that the analytical perspective is mostly used by medical staff, whilst the intuitive perspective is predominantly used by nursing staff.

Cioffi (1997) notes that in the past, nurses (often female), who used their intuitive judgements, may not have been popular with medical (often male) colleagues, who were roused from their beds to a sick service user who had no criteria-related signs or symptoms. This resonates with Benner and Tanner's (1987) previous observation, that medical staff devalue intuitive judgement, however they also point out that some nurses may also share this view. Cioffi (1997) goes on to say that this devaluing may lead individuals to play down the use of intuition because of fear of ridicule. King and McLeod Clark (2002) also recognise this, and note that some student nurses fear being thought silly or stupid if they report their intuitive feelings about a service user in their care. So why should this be? Perry (2000) offers some insight on this aspect, in her exploration of intuition.

Perry (2000: 142) points out that, for her, intuitive understanding is not based on 'specific analysis of substantive data' or 'cause and effect' or 'cognitive processes'. She discusses the issue of how intuition may be brought to bear in the absence of knowing a service user, for example their details, history, illness, etc. and/or in the absence of service user interaction. Therefore, the intuitive practitioner can engage with a degree of rapidity in seeing the service user as a person rather than merely as the service user. Callaghan (2007) makes the point that intuitive practice may not just be part of expert practice, but that non-experts may also have this level of judgement. If this is true, this could have a bearing on all health and social care professionals' views of intuitive practice and judgements. There might be an element of professional jealousy creeping in here, and, rather than acknowledging this, intuitive practitioners (be they expert or non-expert, male or female) are swiftly condemned as being unscientific.

This raises the question of what exactly it is that the practitioner is responding to when they engage in intuitive practice. A research study undertaken by Tveiten et al. (2005) on a group of Norwegian public health nurses (equivalent to the United Kingdom's health visitors) noted that they visited service users (labelling it a 'supervision strategy') as a result of having a 'gut feeling' about the person or family. The nurses reported that they were able to sense whether a child was being adequately cared for or had developmental needs.

This gut feeling was also identified in an earlier study carried out by McCutcheon and Pincombe (2001). They used a Delphi technique and grounded theory to investigate intuition. Their findings yielded that intuition was not something that just happened, but a combination of knowledge, experience and expertise, plus 'personality, environment, acceptance of intuition as a valid "behaviour" and the presence or absence of a nurse/service user relationship' (McCutcheon and Pincombe, 2001: 345). They formulated a model whereby knowledge, experience and expertise brought about synergy, which in turn produced a somatic response or feeling. This feeling, they state, could be either a physical or mental response, occurring at the same time as or shortly after an intuitive event. This somatic sensation has similarly been recorded by Smith et al. (2004), who found a combination of factors that made up intuition in student nurses. These were personal body awareness and an emotional awareness, noting feelings such as apprehension and premonition, in addition to feelings of reassurance. Also, it was found that the two awareness concepts were combined with an ability to make connections, such as reading cues, sensing energy and identifying spiritual connections. What affected the nurse as to whether they acted on these feelings comes back to the environment in which they worked, that is, intuitive practice was either validated (through positive responses by others) or inhibited (through negative responses and devaluing). The McCutcheon and Pincombe (2001) study noted that experienced nurses thought that student nurses were not intuitive, and that male nurses were less intuitive than females; however, when these groups were asked about intuitive practice, both groups reported experiencing such episodes.

Concluding views on intuition

What becomes apparent from reading the literature on intuition is that, first, it is a difficult phenomenon to define. Secondly, there appears to be a division between the use of intuitive practice at an expert level and at a non-expert level. The expert will cite that intuition is built on levels of knowledge and experience, whilst the non-expert reacts to a gut feeling that something is not right. To this end, it could be proposed that the former is 'informed intuition', whilst the latter is 'reactive intuition'. The differences between the two are illustrated in Box 5.1.

Box 5.1   Informed intuition and reactive intuition

Informed intuition

- Significant clinical experience in field
- Prior knowledge and learning
- Understanding the relationship between bio-psycho-social-spiritual aspects and effect on the health of the individual
- Understanding of disease processes
- Ability to identify saliency
- Decision-making ability
- Ability to remember and recall previous experiences
- Proximity to service user
- Able to identify 'at risk' service users
- Assertive behaviours adopted
- Inter-rater agreement

Reactive intuition

- Personal and individual
- Attunement to feelings: 'gut feeling', 'hunch', 'sixth sense'
- Variable clinical experiences
- Uncertain knowledge base
- May be no proximity to service user
- Belief that an event may or will occur

This is echoed in the story of the teaching colleague mentioned earlier and assists with explaining the results that were gained when debating intuition with students and trained staff. However, regardless of the type of intuition brought into play, both need to operate in an environment where it is valued rather than derided. Consequently, senior staff have a significant role to play in helping students identify and respond to moments of intuition, in order to improve judgements on service user care.

Mentorship and Patronage

Unless the future generations of health and social care professionals are knowledgeable in regard to values-based care, then this concept will not take root and flourish. Not only does the ethos of this style of care need to be promoted through the channels of education (discussed in Chapter 7) but, also, because of the nature of health and social care, it requires practice in practice settings. This can best be tackled through a system of mentorship and patronage which embraces the ideals of professional judgement, a prerequisite of values-based care. Education for health and social care professionals already uses a system of mentorship within practice placements, with experienced professionals overseeing and supporting students and less experienced colleagues. This is an ideal portal from which to reinforce the education and promotion of values-based care through practice experience. In addition, patronage, which is generally regarded as the support, encouragement and financial aid that one person or organisation bestows upon another, can also be harnessed to promote the ethos of values-based care through provision of support and finance for schemes of education and training.

Mentorship

It is recognised that mentoring is an effective tool in raising morale and performance generally within health and social care services (Bayley et al., 2004). Within mentorship, a relationship of support is developed between the mentor and mentee, with the mentor working closely with their charge in order to develop both professional and personal skills. This relationship is particularly helpful when mentees are facing new challenges, due, in part, to the strong professional bond which ideally develops between the two colleagues, enabling open and frank discussions to take place. Mentors are normally experienced health or social care professionals who work with and support students or less experienced members of their profession in clinical and other practice areas (Foster-Turner, 2005).

The system of mentorship in health and social care education is already well established for students in practice settings and current mentors can assist student performance by supporting the development of values-based care. However, the mentor system can also be extended to support established workers who have not been educated in values-based care delivery. All health and social care workers need to embrace values-based care as the principal standard for health and social care delivery, leading to an appreciation that evidence-based care is an important aspect in a range of caring skills. Mentors can use a behaviour modification approach (discussed further in Chapter 7) with mentees who are established health and social care workers educated in evidence-based care (as opposed to students of the professions), in order to bring about the recognition, acceptance and practice of values-based care.

During their education, students of the health and social care professions will require a solid, powerful introduction to values-based care, which will include the importance of evidence-based care and how this is incorporated into the holistic approach of values-based care. Mentors, who are often strong role models for students (Stromei, 2000), can demonstrate this personalised, inclusive style of care themselves and discuss its application with their student charges. Students, through education, observation and practice, will then absorb and understand the nuances of this style of care and naturally emulate this in their own field of practice. Thus, the leap from purely evidence-based, service user centred care, which is at present the dominant philosophy in the field of health and social care, to the more inclusive values-based, person-centred approach will occur transitionally as students become qualified and go on to mentor students themselves.

Mentoring has the advantage of being an individualised activity with mentors often working in a one-to-one situation with their charges (Foster-Turner, 2005). Being a personalised approach, it is an ideal way in which to develop in students the knowledge and skills for effective delivery of values-based care, with mentors encouraging students to reflect upon their practice and explore within themselves the effectiveness of their role. Values-based care not only includes respect for the values of service users, it also encompasses the development of personal and professional values for health and social care professionals (Cuthbert and Quallington, 2008). Whilst these values may be discussed, encouraged and explored with students in the academic setting, it will be in practice, through the encouragement and praise of mentors, that students will truly develop and retain these all-important principles, such as trustworthiness, maintaining confidentiality and truthtelling (Cuthbert and Quallington, 2008). Mentors can be encouraged to explore values generally with their charges and to encourage them to reflect upon their personal value base, alongside the purported values of their chosen profession displayed in the relevant codes of practice. The significance of the students' own values in health and social care practice can be discussed in order to encourage deeper levels of analysis and reasoning. This is with the intention of fine-tuning care, in order to provide an individualised service for users which acknowledges opinions and values.

Vignette 5.3 illustrates how mentorship can promote values-based care in practice. The general practitioner, an advocate of values-based decision making, demonstrates to the medical student the ways in which this is practised. In this case, the doctor uses her clinical judgement combined with the service user's beliefs and values to develop a treatment regime to suit this particular service user. Should the service users' beliefs and values contradict a good health outcome, for example, if they were using excessive amounts of alcohol to numb pain, then the doctor would need to explore this with the service user, suggesting alternative treatments and discussing health issues surrounding this.

Vignette 5.3

I recently visited my doctor to discuss a recurrent sore throat which has persisted for the last three months; this is my second visit within this time frame. The doctor had a medical student in the surgery with her and she asked my permission for the student to observe the consultation, which I granted. The doctor asked me if I had been taking medication for my recurrent throat infection since my last visit. I explained that I am an advocate of complementary medicines and have been taking a homeopathic remedy prescribed by a local homeopath, however, although I consider that my throat condition has improved somewhat, it continues to be sore and inflamed. The doctor explained to the student that she likes to work in partnership with her service users and respects their values and beliefs – in my case a belief in complementary medicine. With my permission the doctor took a swab from my throat which she explained she would send for analysis in order to prescribe the correct antibiotics, as the last course of medication did not appear to improve my condition. Meantime, she advised me to continue with my homeopathic remedy and the lemon and honey drinks that I have been taking to ease the inflammation and to visit again in one week's time when the results from the swab would be available.

(Continued)

(Continued)

I find it very reassuring that my doctor listens to my ideas and respects my opinions. I feel that I work in partnership with my doctor in both diagnosing and treating my conditions. Due to this, I consider that I value and respect my doctor's opinions and comply with treatments far more readily than with previous doctors I have encountered. I think that the student working with this doctor will also learn these skills through observation and practice under the mentorship of my doctor who is an experienced clinician.

Patronage

The delivery of health and social care affects all citizens and is, therefore, of importance to everybody. Health and social care workers are employed in a variety of fields from industry to the community and it is essential that educational updates are offered to workers across this spectrum. Programmes of education and training are often expensive to access, however, and if values-based care is to be firmly established then these need to become mandatory for all workers in this field. Corporate or institutional patronage in regard to the sponsorship of values-based care could assist in providing funding and access to courses in this important topic, thus ensuring equity of care delivery across the sectors. However, in a national climate where the provision of health and social care is closely connected to the issue of limited resources, this will not be an easy task. Success could be secured by the wholehearted acceptance of this approach to care by government who could then work closely with partner agencies, such as the voluntary and independent sectors, in order to ensure the promotion of values-based care.

The present environment in health and social care reveals a State which is gradually withdrawing from front-line commitment to delivering services, instead placing a greater emphasis on the workings of a free market economy and on the 'payment of individuals' principle of economic rationalism (Burke, 2000). This philosophy is an echo of the 18th-century concept of the civil society with the recent emergence of the presently rather vague concept of the 'third way' as an alternative to the concept of the State versus free market individualism (Tritter et al., 2003). Patronage of health and social care education fits neatly into this new ethos as it utilises both State and independent sectors in taking responsibility for care provision and, as a consequence, care worker education. This is not a new concept; the independent sector has long been involved in delivering care services as exampled in the following quotation:

Since 2004 UK charity Marie Curie Delivering Choice Programme has worked with doctors and nurses in hospitals, hospices and community services to give people in Lincolnshire with terminal illnesses the choice of dying at home, rather than in hospital ... The King's Fund's analysis of the impact and costs of the programme concludes that it represents a cost effective model of care that can make choosing to die at home a real option for dying patients. (Marie Curie Cancer Care, 2008)

Values-based care would need to be introduced to health and social care workers using a three-tier approach. Students of the health and social care professions could be introduced to this during their education programme and then supported in practice through the mentorship network, as discussed previously. In addition, workers who are already engaged in health and social care delivery could be introduced to values-based care through workshops, giving the possibility to train staff intensively over a few days, thus minimising disruption to the workplace. The third tier of promoting values-based care could consist of regular (preferably annual) updates which would refresh staff knowledge and skills and ensure up-to-date practices are dispersed.

Patronage by government, voluntary and independent agencies could sustain this three-tier support system by funding educational programmes and encouraging uptake of these by the staff involved in care delivery and education and training. Presently, the programmes of education for health and social care professionals are government-led through National Occupational Standards (Skills for Justice, 2009) and the inclusion of values-based care can be made mandatory within these curricula, thus ensuring that the future generations of health and social care workers are knowledgeable in the practice of this holistic style of care. Values-based updates could also be included in professional development programmes as all health and social care professionals need to continually update their knowledge and skills to ensure currency of expertise and competence to practise. Natural dissemination of the concept will also occur through academic journals, books and professional conferences.

Institutional and corporate patronage could support the symbiotic approach to education and training of health and social care staff which synergises both the academic and practice settings. The macro level could consist of patronage for education, training and updates, whilst the micro level could consist of individual support by qualified staff who have been educated in this care delivery philosophy and offered through mentorship programmes.

Vignette 5.4 demonstrates individualised patronage of values-based care in a social care setting. Through education in this new health care policy, the manager clearly sees the benefit to service users of care which embraces both their values and those of the care professionals and thus advocates education and training in values-based care for all staff in this setting.

Vignette 5.4

I am the manager of a day centre run by a charity for the elderly; it is a busy centre and caters for 60 older persons from Monday through to Friday each week. I am undertaking a part-time Diploma in Management of Health and Social Care Services which is being funded by the charity. Part of my course has involved learning about the importance of values-based care and how evidence-based practice fits within this framework. I am aware that my staff have not been trained in values-based care, and this concerns me as I consider that this person-centred approach could benefit my service users by improving the provision of care which they receive. Due to this unease, I am applying for funding from the charity in order that staff at the centre can attend workshops on values-based care which are being offered by the local further education college within my area.

Conclusion

In conclusion, this chapter has discussed how the professional judgement of practitioners is a crucial factor in delivering optimum care to service users. This judgement, which is a combination of expertise and intuition, is honed through professional practice and reflection on the various experiences this provides. Values-based care delivers health and social care that is bespoke to each service user, recognising and accepting individuality and diversity and embracing the importance of professional judgement. Evidence-based practice is an important component of values-based care and it is recommended that the present educational and clinical emphasis on this important aspect of care delivery continues alongside the promotion of values-based health and social care. Programmes of education sponsored by patronage from various health and social care providers and benefactors, and clinical experience reinforced by an effective network of mentorship, can promote the practice of values-based care. These are time-honoured strategies and, therefore, essential requisites in implementing this new and improved model of care delivery. It is no longer enough to talk about embracing service user diversity and individuality and yet provide care that is, in essence, dictated and uniform to all. Recognition of the importance of values-based care has already begun and this must be exploited in order to optimise health and social care services for all.

References

Banning, M. (2007) 'A review of clinical decision-making models and current research', *Journal of Clinical Nursing*, 17(2): 187–95.

Bayley, H., Chambers, R. and Donovan, C. (2004) *The Good Mentoring Toolkit for Healthcare*. Oxford: Radcliffe.

Benner, P. (1984) *From Novice to Expert: Excellence and Power in Clinical Nursing Practice*. Menlo Park, CA: Addison-Wesley.

Benner, P. and Tanner, C. (1987) 'How expert nurses use intuition', *American Journal of Nursing*, 87(1): 23–31.

Benner, P., Tanner, C. and Chesla, C. (1996) *Expertise in Nursing Practice: Caring, Clinical Judgement and Ethics*. New York: Springer.

Buetow, S. and Kenealy, T. (2000) 'Evidence-based medicine: the need for a new definition', *Journal of Evaluation in Clinical Practice*, 6(2): 85–91.

Burke, D. (2000) 'Economic rationalism in health and education: impact on the academic physician', *Internal Medicine Journal*, 30(1): 71–4.

Callaghan, L. (2007) 'Advanced nursing practice: an idea whose time has come', *Journal of Clinical Nursing*, 17(2): 205–13.

Cioffi, J. (1997) 'Heuristics, servants to intuition, in clinical decision-making', *Journal of Advanced Nursing*, 26: 203–8.

Colyer, H. and Kamath, P. (1999) 'Evidence-based practice. A philosophical and political analysis: some matters for consideration by professional practitioners', *Journal of Advanced Nursing*, 29: 188–93.

Cuthbert, S. and Quallington, J. (2008) *Health and Social Care Theory and Practice: Values for Care Practice*. Devon: Reflect Press Ltd.

Dennett, D.C. (2005) 'Cognitive wheels: the frame problem of AI', in A. Barber (2006) *Reading 6: Language and Thought. Course Book 3 – Thought and Experience: Themes in the Philosophy of Mind (Course AA308)*, pp. 217–23. Milton Keynes: Open University Press.

Dowie, R.S. and Macnaughton, J. (2000) *Clinical Judgement Evidence in Practice*. Oxford: Oxford University Press.

Effken, J.A. (2001) 'Informational basis for expert tuition', *Journal of Advanced Nursing*, 34: 246–55.

Fish, D. and Coles, C. (eds) (1998) *Developing Professional Judgement in Health and Social Care: Learning through the Critical Appreciation of Practice*. Oxford: Butterworth-Heinemann.

Foster-Turner, J. (2005) *Coaching and Mentoring in Health and Social Care*. Oxford: Radcliffe.

Harbison, J. (1991) 'Clinical decision making in nursing', *Journal of Advanced Nursing*, 16: 404–7.

King, L. and McCleod Clark, J. (2002) 'Intuition and the development of expertise in surgical ward and intensive care nurses', *Journal of Advanced Nursing*, 37: 322–9.

Leddy, S. and Pepper, J.M. (1993) *Conceptual Bases of Professional Nursing*, 3rd edition. Philadelphia, PA: Lippincott, Williams and Wilkins.

Luntley, M. (2007) 'Care, sensibility and judgement', in J.S. Drummond and P. Standish (eds) *The Philosophy of Nurse Education*. Basingtoke: Palgrave Macmillan, pp. 77–90.

Marie Curie Cancer Care (2008) *Dying patients given greater choice to die at home at no extra cost to the NHS, King's Fund report concludes*. Available at: http://deliveringchoice.mariecurie.org.uk/news_and_events/press_releases/kings-fund-report.htm [accessed 1 December 2009]

Melnyk, B.M. and Fineout-Overholt, E. (2005) *Evidence-based Practice in Nursing and Healthcare*. Philadelphia, PA: Lippincott, Williams and Wilkins.

McCutcheon, H.H.I. and Pincombe, J. (2001) 'Intuition: an important tool in the practice of nursing', *Journal of Advanced Nursing*, 35: 342–8.

Pearson, A., Field, J. and Jordon, Z. (2007) *Evidence-based Clinical Practice in Nursing and Health and Social Care: Assimilating Research, Experience and Expertise*. Oxford: Blackwell.

Perry, M.A. (2000) 'Reflections on intuition and expertise', *Journal of Clinical Nursing*, 9: 137–45.

Petrova, M., Dale, J. and Fulford, K.W.M. (2006) 'Values-based practice in primary care: easing the tensions between individual values, ethical principles and best evidence', *British Journal of General Practice*, 56: 703–9.

Rashotte, J. and Carnevale, F.A. (2004) 'Medical and nursing clinical decision making: a comparative epistemological analysis', *Nursing Philosophy*, 5: 60–74.

Sackett, D.L., Richardson, W.S., Rosenberg, W. and Haynes, R.B. (1997) *Evidence-based Medicine: What it is and What it isn't*. London: Churchill Livingstone.

Savage, P. (1993) 'Ethical boundaries', *Senior Nurse*, 13(3): 5–6.

Schön, D.A. (1983) *The Reflective Practitioner: How Professionals Think in Action*. New York: Basic Books.

Schön, D.A. (1987) *Educating the Reflective Practitioner*. San Francisco: Jossey-Bass.

Schön, D.A. (1991) *The Reflective Practitioner: How Professionals Think in Action*, 2nd edition. London: Basic Books.

Skills for Justice (2009) *What are NOS?* Available at: www.skillsforjustice. com/template01.asp?pageid=37 [accessed 1 December 2009]

Smith, A.J., Thurkettle, M.A. and de la Cruz, F.A. (2004) 'Use of intuition by nursing students: instrument development and testing', *Journal of Advanced Nursing*, 47: 614–22.

Stromei, L.K. (2000) 'Increasing retention and success through mentoring', *New Directions for Community Colleges*, 2002(112): 55–62.

Tritter, J.Q., Barley, V., Daykin, N., Evans, S., McNeill, J., Rimmer, J., Sanidas, M. and Turton, P. (2003) 'Divided care and the Third Way: user involvement in statutory and voluntary sector cancer services', *Sociology of Health and Illness*, 25(5): 429–56.

Tveiten, S., Ellefsen, B. and Severinsson, E. (2005) 'Conducting service user supervision in community health and social care', *International Journal of Nursing Practice*, 11: 68–76.

Woodbridge, K. and Fulford, K.W.M. (2004) *Whose Values? A Workbook for Values-based Practice in Mental Health and Social Care*. London: Sainsbury Centre for Mental Health.

6 The Value and Values of Service Users

Annette McIntosh, Julie Dulson and
Julie Bailey-McHale.
Vignettes by Joanne Greenwood

In this chapter, service user involvement in health and social care is explored with a focus on the values underpinning this concept. The first section concerns the current context of service user involvement and the nature and challenges of partnership working. A key initiative in collaborative working, that of the service user as an expert, is critically analysed in the next section and the chapter moves to a conclusion with a discussion of diversity and a call for not merely acknowledging, but celebrating, the difference and diversity evident within the values of individuals.

Service user Involvement and the Characteristics and Challenges of Effective Partnership Working

On a general level, the concept of respecting the values of individuals has long been a central tenet for health and social care professionals in their delivery of care. As Warne and McAndrew (2008) noted, it is important that there is a clear understanding of what it is that individuals value about their lives, requiring care givers to be open to, and non-judgemental about, others' opinions and points of view. However, while the notion of placing individuals fully at the centre of their care and ensuring that their opinions are heard, valued and acted upon has been advocated in the health and social care professions for many years, in reality it is only in the past decade or so that the full importance of service user involvement has received due attention.

Service users can be involved in care provision in a number of ways and on a number of levels, as will be discussed later in the chapter. As Bradshaw (2008) stated, service improvement can be realised through personalised care, partnership working in decision making, offering service users choice and information, securing the participation of users in policy making and enhancing care options through provider contestability.

This need for the full involvement of service users in their care is now recognised internationally, especially evident in America, Australia, New Zealand and Japan. In the UK, the Department of Health (DH) has highlighted the importance of the role of service user involvement in a range of policy documents such as *The NHS Plan* (DH, 2000), *Involving Patients and the Public in Health Care* (DH, 2002a) and *Creating a Patient Led NHS* (DH, 2005). Recent DH publications further set out the requirements for the health and social care professions in relation to involving service users in their care. In the publication, *Implementation of the Right to Choice and Information Set Out in the NHS Constitution*, the new rights of service users (interestingly, still called patients here by the DH) are detailed, including the right to make choices about their care underpinned by information to support these choices (DH, 2009a). In another guidance document, the DH addresses the commissioning of personalised care planning which, while primarily concerned with long-term conditions, is noted to be applicable generally (DH, 2009b). In this, the need for health and social care professionals to ensure that people and their carers are equal partners in care planning is highlighted, with an emphasis on supporting individuals to have their say. In addition, it is recognised that the process of planning in health and social care should be negotiated and led by the individual, in a process that takes into account the service user's goals, strengths, wishes and aspirations. The notion that the choices individuals make at a micro level should be aggregated and fed in at a macro level to influence commissioning decisions and patterns for the larger population is also recommended to the professions (DH, 2009b).

The Department of Health (2009b) noted that while there were many areas of effective working in areas of health and social care including community matrons, children's community nurses and social care professionals, there was a need for the approach of service user involvement to be embedded far more widely. The effective participation of service users has been addressed in some other areas beside those cited by the DH. These include care of the elderly (Andrews et al., 2004; McCormack, 2003), cancer and palliative care (Evans et al., 2003), mental health (Hui and Stickley, 2007; Lester et al., 2006; Peterson et al., 2008; Stickley, 2008), learning disability (Young and Chesson, 2006) and health and social care education (Felton and Stickley,

2004; Forrest et al., 2000). The DH (2007) noted that full participation from the professions was essential in order to bring about placing the service user at the core of service delivery, and recommended that local forums, task groups and networks were established, involving staff and service users as active participants to bring about the change.

For partnership working to be effective, there are various characteristics that are recognised as being essential. Coulter (1999) stated that while the professional is knowledgeable about the individuals' condition, only service users and carers know about their experiences, circumstances, habits, preferences and values; the partnership approach to care should be based on mutual respect. This notion of an equal and dynamic partnership is reiterated by the DH (2009b) who recommended that the process of partnership working should focus on negotiating and deciding outcomes that the individual and their carer want to achieve, is owned by them and which promote joined-up working, especially between health and social care.

The recent Darzi report (DH, 2008) highlighted the values contained in the new NHS Constitution regarding service users and their carers. These included the premise that each individual is valued as a person and that their aspirations and commitments in life are respected, with their priorities, needs, abilities and limits being recognised. This mirrors the views of McCormack (2003) who considered that respecting values is at the core of individualised care, with the requirement for professionals to understand what people value about their life and how they make sense of their circumstances. Evans et al. (2003) highlighted the need for flexible and timely access to information being required to assist individuals in making choices and also noted that communication was an important factor in encouraging service user involvement. When considering the role of service user involvement in education, Felton and Stickley (2004) highlighted the need for an infrastructure to fully underpin the process, support from those in education and a balancing of the power inequalities (perceived or real) that can exist in partnership working. Forrest et al. (2000) opined that service users, educationalists and students require support and preparation for their roles, with the service users additionally receiving appropriate remuneration for their contributions. Sawyer (2005) encapsulated all the elements and characteristics of true partnership working, in which there is mutual trust, stating that this requires: open communication; shared values and goals; shared risk; sharing and solving problems; and a no-blame culture.

Whilst there are thus many essential components for effective partnership working, there are equally many challenges that have to be overcome. The

DH (2009b) noted that, in advocating a partnership approach to care, a less paternalistic approach was required, with the adoption of a more empowering ethos. This echoes the sentiments expressed by Coulter (1999) who considered that while paternalism was endemic in the NHS, it should have no place in modern health care and that a move to meaning-ful partnership working was overdue. Similarly, in the DH (2007) publi-cation, *Putting People First – A Shared Vision and Commitment to the Transformation of Adult Social Care*, the ideals of replacing paternalistic, reactive care of variable quality with a future system where individuals have the maximum control and power over the services they require and want, is emphasised, with the right to self-determination seen as being at the core of a reformed system of service planning and delivery. Sawyer (2005), writing about embedding service user-driven outcomes in domi-ciliary care, considered that one of the greatest challenges lay in bring-ing about the necessary culture change to achieve this effectively. The DH (2002b) publication, *Shifting the Balance of Power – The Next Steps*, also stipulated the need for behaviour change with a greater focus on team working and enabling and supporting people, and less control and hierar-chical patterns of delivery. As Bradshaw (2008) reflected, the prevailing policy drivers mean that the time-honoured knowledge and wisdom of the professions will become increasingly scrutinised and questioned and pro-vide challenges to be overcome, especially to the medical profession. It has been noted that changing the long-established views, values and behav-iours of health and social care professionals will require support from all levels, alongside the development of staff (DH, 2002b).

The need for leadership to ensure that the involvement of service users is not tokenistic but valued is widely recognised and embedded within the policy drivers. The DH (2007), whilst recognising some cutting-edge work, stated that national and local leadership would be necessary, alongside a shared com-mitment to social justice, not only for embedding the changes required for a system transformation, but also to address the demographic realities inherent in affecting such a change. The DH (2009b) opined that the cultural change required to fully embed service user involvement at a local level had often not been underpinned by full support and leadership at management level.

Coulter (1999) considered that several other hurdles needed to be overcome to ensure safe and effective partnership working, including the preparation and readiness of service users to assume responsibility for decision making. Research by Litva et al. (2002) indicated that there were variations in public willingness to be involved in health care decisions and noted that, while there was a strong desire for involvement at system and programme levels, there was less willingness to be involved at the individual level. Two issues were identified as being important for full participation: the need for information and the need to consider the experiences and emotions of individuals.

The realities of involving service users to benefit and enhance the education of health and social care professionals, including involvement in the design and delivery of curricula, have also been noted to pose difficulties. These included the often conflicting views and values of educationalists and service users, ensuring appropriate representativeness and avoiding tokenism (Forrest et al., 2000). In addition, Felton and Stickley (2004) stated that failure to address the disempowerment of service users was challenging, considering that this required a shift in power that in turn can result in the educationalists feeling disempowered and justifying the status quo, instead of fully embracing the involvement of service users.

The general and fundamental requirement for adequate resourcing to fully implement service user involvement at all levels has also received attention in the literature. An example of the concern surrounding this issue comes from Newman et al. (2008) who considered that whilst social care has a reputation for leading the way with service user initiatives, often serving as models for other services, the reality is that the profession could start to lag behind because of a lack of resources; they warn that tightening resources could lead to the voice of service users being squeezed out.

Notwithstanding these challenges and concerns, it is evident that the move towards a meaningful involvement of service users, with full recognition of their individual values, is gaining momentum. Relatively recent initiatives include the holding by service users of individualised, or personalised, budgets with which they can decide how they will meet their health or social care needs. Sawyer (2008) noted that in social work, personal budgets, while only one part of the move towards self-directed support and individualised care, were implemented to empower individuals to choose the services they felt met their needs and priorities; the use of brokers to help guide service users and their families is increasingly being used.

Service users are also becoming increasingly influential in health and social care research. For example, in a qualitative study exploring mental health recovery in Scotland, service users were part of the steering group and also recruited as interviewers (Brown and Kandirikirira, 2007). The findings of the research showed that for those service users who were involved in service user groups and campaigns, the experience was a positive one and helped their recovery. Further, Brown and Kandirikirira's study highlighted that some of the participants believed that 'service users were the unrecognised experts in the field of mental health whose opinions need to be more valued' (2007: 36).

Service users' and carers' participation in shaping and influencing health and social care is multi-faceted; the next section explores consumer roles and the concept of expert service users working synergistically with professionals.

Service Users as Consumers and Expert Patients

The rise of service user involvement in health and social care provision is often linked to the development of consumerism in the 1980s (Edwards, 2000). Rush (2004) argues that user involvement is best understood through a historical context and while Rush's (2004) paper specifically focuses upon user involvement in mental health settings, reflecting upon the social and political thinking of the time is important to the context of user involvement in all health and social care settings. One of the earliest examples of user groups, the 'Friends of Alleged Lunatics Society', led by John Perceval, campaigned for compassionate care in the asylums in the 18th century. The contextualisation of mental health care was at the time changing from a model of moral degeneracy towards a model of moral management led by Pinel in France and Tuke at the York Retreat (Rush, 2004). Central to the model of moral management was the idea that mental illness could be alleviated and in some instances cured by providing the person with a caring environment (Rush, 2004). Later, the 1950s saw the advent of psychiatric medications which reinforced the concept of the medical model of health and the notion of 'doctor knows best' which negated the need for user involvement and reinforced the concept of paternalism as an influential barrier to user involvement. Consumerism brought with it the notion of choice, placing the individual in receipt of care at its centre. However, consumerism is often criticised in that choice is only useful if the choices available are acceptable to those requiring the services. Consumerism has led to a large increase in the service user movement (Felton and Stickley, 2004) and, in recent years, service users have developed themselves into a forceful social movement, often actively influencing aspects of care such as the availability and prescribing of medicines. It is apparent that user involvement is a central facet of conventional health and social care and this is evidenced by initiatives such as the expert patient programme. Whilst it is possible to be critical of the expert patient programme, it is important to acknowledge that this national initiative clearly places user involvement within the mainstream of health services and so demonstrates the change in focus of health and social care delivery.

The concept of the expert patient programme was first introduced in the DH's white paper *Our Healthier Nation – Saving Lives* (DH, 1999). A further DH paper in 2001 set out the vision that expert patient programmes would become part of the standard provision of the NHS and this was further reiterated in the NHS health improvement plan (DH, 2004) which stated that the expert patient programme would be available in all Primary Care Trusts within four years. The underpinning philosophy of the expert patient is that those experiencing chronic health conditions represent an untapped resource, both for their own health and the health of others experiencing similar conditions. The suggestion is that health providers will empower those with long-term health conditions to not only self-manage their condition, but also to support others to self-manage through the expert patient programme. This programme consists of a number of taught sessions, delivered by lay persons who themselves are suffering from a chronic condition, regarding self-management techniques and, in simple terms, involves service users educating other service users.

At first glance, the concept of the expert patient appears to be a clear step in the right direction towards a more user-led health service and so should be welcomed. However, it is important to examine the underpinning philosophies of the expert patient to identify if this programme will indeed strengthen the cause of user involvement in services. The most evident consideration is the name of the programme: 'the expert patient'. It is widely recognised that use of language is a key strategy used to define roles and reinforce status of individuals (Sang, 2004). Much of the literature regarding user involvement in services highlights the importance of professionals utilising a respectful language that is value-free. The Oxford English Dictionary (2009) defines a patient as 'a person receiving or registered to receive medical treatment'. This term implies a passive role, a person in receipt of care rather than an equal partner in that care. Failure to address power differentials between service users and health professionals is frequently cited as a barrier to service user involvement (Poulton, 1999) and the use of the term patient in the title of this initiative appears to reinforce rather than address those differentials.

The title of expert, according to Wilson (2001), is usually used when describing someone who has undergone applicable training and further study and so is indicative of increased status and knowledge. Tang and Anderson (1999) suggested that the idea of an expert is further reinforced by the process of socialisation. The person is viewed as an expert and so their opinion is seen as that of an expert, which further reinforces their status as an expert. However, Robert et al. (2003) argued that many health professionals find it difficult to view service users as experts and so this process of sociali-sation will not occur. The arguments in the literature regarding the repre-sentativeness of service users is a key example of this – professionals inhibit service user involvement through the suggestion that a service user can only represent their own views or the views of their own kind, that is people with a similar condition, and as it is not possible to include everyone with differing health problems, it is best not to try. Professionals often forget, however, that they themselves are trying to be the voice of all other professionals.

Further, according to Tang and Anderson (1999), a person will be una-ble to achieve expert status until they have access to equal rights and equal resources. A report by Squire and Hill (2006), both members of the Patient Experience team which worked with the DH to set up the expert patients programme, suggests, although does not explicitly state, that many of the users who delivered the expert patient programme were unpaid volunteers, highlighting a fundamental disparity when compared with professionals working on the programme. Robert et al. (2003) suggested that expecting service users to contribute their time for free demonstrates a clear lack of recognition for the value of the service users' contribution and is a clear bar-rier to effective user involvement which must be addressed.

Hickey and Kipping (1998) suggested that user involvement in services should be considered on a continuum with information giving at one end through consultation, partnership and finally user control at the other. Infor-mation giving involves solely the provision of information regarding services or treatment to users; consultation builds upon this and requires service pro-viders to seek the views of service users regarding services, but does not nec-essarily mean that those views will be addressed and that changes will occur as a result of the consultation. The partnership approach requires service users and providers to have equal standing (and equal power) and decisions to be made jointly. To ensure this approach is effective, it is necessary that all parties have access to the same information and the same abilities for inter-preting that information. The final approach is that of user control – here the power is fully redistributed to the users. The user, or group of users, will make the decision whether or not to involve others in the decision-making process. Some decisions will affect only the individual user, such as suita-bility and timing of treatments, whereas other decisions may affect a whole group of users, such as provision of a service. In this case, it will be necessary to decide whose needs are paramount in the case of conflict.

Equipping service users with the knowledge and skills to manage their own health and to assist others is, one could argue, suggestive of user-controlled services. However, Hickey and Kipping (1998) further suggested that the amount of involvement a user of services can have in those services will be dependent upon their power to influence decisions. In this case, the power to influence could be considered in terms of knowledge. The premise of the expert patient programme is that service users will be empowered to self-manage their condition and to train others to do so. However, the question remains about who exactly will decide what information will be given to the service users during their training. It is not clear from the literature how differences in opinion regarding the information provided are to be managed or resolved. The national evaluation of the pilot of the expert patient programme found that some participants were unhappy at having to adhere to a fixed script whilst delivering the programme which suggests that those involved in the delivery felt they had more to offer than the constraints of the programme allowed. It further suggests that the programme had been written without the participation of those who were delivering it, which is suggestive of the lowest level of Hickey and Kippings' (1998) user-involvement continuum, that of information giving.

The origins for the expert patient programme come from Lorig et al.'s (1996) chronic disease self-management programme, which originated in the USA (DH, 1999). This programme focuses education and training on 12 tasks which Lorig et al. (1996) suggested are common to all chronic disease sufferers. These tasks include monitoring symptoms, maintaining an adequate diet, communicating with health professionals, not smoking and using medications. Pre-determining the information which those experiencing chronic illnesses require and providing only that information does, according to Sang (2004), evoke images of paternalism and further widens the power imbalance between health professional and service user. The 12 tasks also appear to reinforce the notion of a medical model of illness. Wilson et al. (2007) agree, suggesting that the content of the expert patient programme reinforces the medical perspective of chronic illness. This is suggestive of the idea then that the aim of the programme is to increase service users' compliance with medically determined interventions, an aim which Lewis (2003) argues is paradoxical to the philosophy of service user involvement.

It is clear that service users are likely to base their decisions regarding treatment options on the information provided to them by health care professionals. Although the information given during the expert patient programme is not delivered by professionals, as it is based upon the medical model, it will mirror the advice from the professionals and will in turn be provided by those who, through the title of the programme, are deemed to be experts. This further reinforces the notion that the expert patient programme is merely a way of promoting compliance with medical approaches. Nash-Wong (2006) suggested that self-management programmes can develop what she termed 'super consumers'. These are service users who have the knowledge to not only identify when they are unwell but also to know what type of treatment to request from their doctor. Nash-Wong (2006) suggested that pharmaceutical companies should utilise the opportunities afforded by self-management programmes and work to ensure that the information provided complements, or even includes, their own brand products. The prospect that self-management programmes, and therefore the expert patient programme, can be manipulated, not only as a tool to increase compliance but also as a marketing ploy by pharmaceutical companies, leads one to question the underpinning philosophy of the initiative, whether it really is about empowerment or more a method of control.

Hickey and Kipping (1998) described two differing philosophies which underpin service user involvement: the consumerist approach and the democratisation approach. According to a consumerist philosophy, the aim of involving users is to seek and identify their views to evaluate the quality of a service. The consumerist approach, which views service users as consumers, became a dominant model of health care delivery during the 1990s and was intended to create an internal market for health care (Rhodes and Nocon, 1998). The opposing philosophy, the democratisation approach, views users not as recipients of care but as citizens within the care community. This means that rather than evaluating the effectiveness of a service, citizens will consider the content of the service or the need for it to even exist.

According to Edwards (2000), it was the dominance of consumerism within health care policy which paved the way for policy regarding user involvement in services. Critics of the consumerist approach suggest that consumerism fosters a tokenistic approach to user involvement by offering a way for users to express their wishes regarding service design, with no real hope of those wishes being realised. The expert patient programme can be seen to be based on consumerist values as it offers a way for service users to take control of their health care, but only within the parameters of the clearly defined health care system. This approach can be summed up as the professional helping the service user to learn to manage their condition in the best way that the professional sees fit; essentially empowering a person to do as they are told, which is surely an oxymoron?

There are, however, clear benefits to the expert patient programme and these should not be minimised. Those involved in the programme benefit from the support of meeting others in a similar position and the hope that the prospect of self-management brings; this is not a case of throwing the baby out with the bathwater. However, whilst the expert patient programme offers opportunities, it is capable of so much more. If we want people to take control of their own lives and health, then surely we should equip them with the skills to do this in whichever way is best for them. The expert patient programme should be less about learning how to agree and comply with health professionals and more about how to identify the most appropriate way to manage the health and well-being of the service user themselves. As will be seen in the next section, this involves not merely acknowledging, but celebrating, the difference and diversity evident within the values of individuals.

Vignette 6.1 demonstrates how even very young service users can become experts in their own health and social care.

Vignette 6.1

I am a qualified nurse and my three-year-old son has suffered from severe eczema from the age of six weeks, constantly experiencing 'flare ups' and although his eczema was well managed at home, it showed no signs of improvement. Throughout this time there were periods of despair, frustration and episodes of severe sleep deprivation for myself and my son, due to lack of any improvement in his skin condition; this resulted in our coping mechanisms diminishing rapidly. All allergy tests at this time showed negative results and the next line of treatment was to be a chemotherapy regime. At this stage I became desperate for any answers to his medical problems. He had previously been treated by a district general hospital and specialist children's hospital but to no avail; essentially I felt that the care for my child was not meeting his, or, indeed, my needs and that we had no power or influence in determining a way forward.

One day whilst reading a nursing journal, I noticed contact details for a nurse consultant in a dermatology unit in a teaching hospital and decided to phone her. She advised me to see my GP and request a referral to a consultant allergist. After discussion with my GP, my son was referred to a consultant dermatologist in a large specialist teaching hospital that evening. I discussed his care with the consultant and agreed a plan for the treatment and care of my son. Throughout the consultations, my child was included in discussions regarding his care and treatment at a level of understanding appropriate for his age group. Therefore, not only were my 'expert views' taken into account, but also those of my son from a very early age. Due to his ongoing health care needs and the partnership that has developed between our family and the healthcare professionals treating him, he has already started on the path of becoming an expert patient from a very young age, as all the decisions made regarding his health care see him at the centre in the decision-making process.

Celebrating Diversity

This section was originally entitled acknowledging diversity. The notion of acknowledging diversity has been accepted for a number of decades now. The initial suggestion for the title did however create a sense of tension at the use of words. Do we remain at the stage of acknowledging diversity, or should we be embracing a new era of diversity, one in which diversity is not merely acknowledged but celebrated? On considering the difference in the two approaches, it occurred to me that there is a distinct and radical difference between acknowledging something and celebrating it. I gladly acknowledge a colleague's birthday with a gesture and an automatic 'happy birthday'. When I celebrate the birthday of my partner, I will consider and prepare for the event and invest time and effort to ensure it is right, thus ensuring that the day and the sentiment is real and meaningful. Could it be, therefore, that, whilst on a professional basis it is relatively easy to acknowledge diversity, it does not require a tremendous amount of effort or commitment? To celebrate diversity puts the professional in a position of affirmation, affirming not just that something is different but that the difference adds something of value, and so should be valued. This is an important concept to appreciate when considering working in partnership with others within health and social care settings; tokenism is an easy trap in which to fall and has been a regular criticism of marginalised groups attempting to find a voice. Valuing individual experience is what transforms good health and social care into excellent care. Valuing individual experience inevitably means that the health and social care professional must see difference and value it for what it is.

The challenges in connecting collaborative practice with a celebration of diversity are immense. Arguably, health and social care professionals have not even begun to adequately incorporate service user involvement effectively, so considering the question of diversity within this debate is complex. The slogan 'the personal is political' was used widely during the 1960s and 1970s by feminists. Part of the power of this slogan comes from the transformation of what is personal, and so private, into the public domain of political activity. The Women's Movement took the personal, diverse experiences of women and made them a subject of legitimate debate. This section explores whether it is possible to take the personal and diverse experiences of the service user and make those experiences truly significant in a personal, professional and political manner.

Diversity can be understood in terms of difference. An important contemporary development has been the establishment of the notion of the politics of difference (Weedon, 1999). It has been suggested that respecting diversity involves a recognition of the intrinsic worth and uniqueness of each individual (Bailey-McHale, 2008). This concept is an important aspect of professional codes of practice (General Social Care Council, 2002; Health Professions Council, 2008; Nursing and Midwifery Council, 2008). Diversity, and respect for difference, are now synonymous with values-based practice. The recognition of difference, rather than the notion of sameness sometimes generated by the notion of equality, is an important development in this area. However, how difference is defined can be loaded with reflections of power relationships within society; difference can be seen in terms of desirable or not desirable.

The advantages of user participation in health and social care are well documented (see previous sections). However, there are criticisms of the approach and clear tensions between professionals and service users. A literature review exploring service user participation in mental health rehabilitation (Peterson et al., 2008) identifies some of these tensions within mental health practice. This literature review demonstrates the differences between service users' perspectives on participation and the perspective of the professional. One particular study reviewed (Lester et al., 2006), demonstrated how general practitioners and nurses were reluctant to involve users of services or to see service users as collaborative partners. Conversely, the review also describes the trend towards valuing more active participation.

What is it about service user involvement that makes it so troublesome? There are undoubtedly practical considerations, not least the questions of who should be involved, how they should be involved and at what level of involvement. Arguably, at the crux of this is the question: where does power lie? The nature of power relations between the professional (those with power) and the service user (without power) becomes essential to deconstruct. It is perhaps only when this is understood that service user involvement will create a more meaningful and effective process of partnership working, a process that leaves service users feeling assured that they have played an active role in the creation of something, rather than merely responding to given agendas (the act of being consulted).

At one level, power can be understood in two distinct ways (Hui and Stickley, 2007). The constant sum concept of power suggests that power is limited; that there is a set amount of power available and if an organisation or profession wants to involve others, then it has to give some of that power away. Power becomes a commodity. Conversely, power can be understood in terms of a non-constant sum approach. Power is not seen as limited but rather as an infinite source. This approach suggests that power can be created in others through a whole range of different activities. The reader is directed to the work of Foucault (1980) who suggested that those with power are able to create a 'truth' associated with their power and social role so recreating significant power relationships that are viewed as normal. These concepts offer an interesting backdrop to the whole question of service user involvement and the incorporation of difference and diversity within this. Foucault (1972) suggested that every discourse has two aspects – power and knowledge – and he was particularly interested in the ways in which power is maintained through language. Within the context of service user involvement, this becomes a critical perspective as the language of those in power serves to reinforce the powerlessness of others. For service users engaging in partnership working, this is a crucial way in which they can be alienated from sometimes complex processes. Very often, service users will lament the overuse of jargon and the ways in which this prevents real and meaningful participation. Those without the necessary vocabulary remain, inevitably, in a position of powerlessness. Hui and Stickley (2007), in their discourse analysis of mental health policy and mental health service user perspectives on involvement, emphasised the difference in the language of government publications regarding involvement, compared to that of service user publications. They identified a difference in perspective within government documents compared to the perspective of the service user. Within the government publications, there were a number of key emerging themes. These included inconsistencies with the language used to refer to service users; the notion of service user involvement and what is meant by that; the nature of power and the notion of a service user-led NHS. The service user perspective emphasised power, control and change; with theory, policy and practice and the service user as expert by experience. The suggestion here is that at a fundamental level, the aspirations of government publications and the aspirations of service users are very different. Another important point, however, is the diversity and differing perspectives that exist within service user organisations and across the range of service users.

What is the way forward for service user involvement in terms of celebrating the diversity that this offers and ensuring real and meaningful participation? In a sense, the answer to this question should come from those who engage with services and want a say in how services should look. One approach would emphasise the continued involvement of service users within consultation panels, as committee members, and within higher education provision. This approach in many ways reflects the situation currently. Service users can be educated as to the appropriate language and customs of Trust boards, universities, professional bodies etc., and can continue to effect change in this way. The second, and arguably the more radical approach, suggests that service users will find real power from the sharing of a collective voice and that by harnessing the power of the collective, real and lasting change can be achieved. The second approach challenges the very basis of how service users are consulted and listened to, and so challenges notions of power and powerlessness. The notion of service user as provider, researcher and educator, not just consumer, may challenge the whole idea of service user involvement. There are, of course, tensions within this approach; there is a danger that it ignores the heterogeneous nature of service user groups. We are a long way from creating systems that truly reflect the diverse nature of service users and their differing priorities and values. Currently, service user involvement is constructed in a way that does not encourage meaningful engagement with the important dimensions of power and inequality, nor do these systems necessarily recognise issues of difference amongst service users.

Service user involvement is now an expectation on both the political and practice agenda. This in itself is a testimony to the resilience of service user activists in many areas of health and social care. This expectation, however, hides some of the tensions and conflicts evident in incorporating full service user participation. At the crux of service user participation are complex power dimensions that, unless acknowledged and explicitly explored, will always undermine meaningful activity. If professionals are to truly involve service users in all aspects of health and social care, they will need to take an honest view of their own capacity to share power and ultimately to share the label of 'expert'. A frame of reference that celebrates this participation, rather than merely acknowledging its usefulness, is needed to ensure the radical and potentially transformative nature of service user participation.

Vignette 6.2 illustrates personal involvement in health and social care services from a service user perspective.

Vignette 6.2

I am a 38-year-old mother of two children, aged five and three years and a nurse by background. For the last ten years I have worked in the field of nurse education and therefore have an understanding of the drive for service user involvement in health care. In my everyday working life this has involved having an awareness of the importance and significance of the role of the service users within the nursing curriculum.

However, on a personal level, my interaction with health care professionals had been minimal and routine. This was to change, however, following the birth of my second child. I attended a six week post natal check where an assessment had been taken to eliminate the possibility of post-natal depression. The score was significantly raised and the health visitor contacted me to discuss her concerns. I was asked if I felt anxious and depressed and I truthfully replied that I did not. Over the months, my symptoms gradually worsened. The main reason I did not seek help at this time was mainly due to personal pride and an overriding sense of failure that I was unable to fight the symptoms myself.

However, the anxiety and depression were severely exacerbated by returning to work and I ended up attending the GP's surgery in a distressed state. The experience I subsequently had was a positive one, with the GP including me in the decisions about my care. I felt that the communication was open and honest and that I was fully consulted about the choices available to me; I felt that there was a mutual trust between myself and the GP. This helped me to make the right choice about my care, further supported by information (verbal and written) which informed my decision making.

The most important decision I had to make was whether or not to take anti-depressants as I was extremely fearful of feeling any worse than I already did and was not keen to start medication. However, explanations were given and timescales set within my own limits, so I felt that I was allowed to take control of the situation. I did feel that allowing me to have a choice regarding my treatments and medications, alongside the collaboration between different members of the multi-disciplinary team, ensured effective, trusting partnerships were established in line with my well-being. However, I recognise that I was perhaps fortunate as I am aware that this does not reflect the experiences of others I know. I feel that the challenges that can sometimes arise perhaps did not in my case, maybe due to my nursing and educational background being valued by the professionals.

Conclusion

The dominant paradigms within health and social care are gradually shifting. The traditional approach, characterised by an authoritative and paternalistic attitude, is becoming less accepted. An emphasis on collaborative, partnership working with service users is much more apparent now; an emphasis on the service user having their say and, in essence, having their values fully valued. This is demonstrated in the chapter's vignettes.

However, the reality is that this is patchy in its execution. Areas of excellence have been recognised, but the challenges involved in ensuring that service user involvement is not tokenistic, but meaningful, has meant that there are still calls for changes in professionals' attitudes and behaviours so that the values and opinions of service users are fully met. Inherent in this is the need to address the concept of often complex power dimensions which can undermine partnership working at every level; these require exploration and acknowledgement of the fact that for true involvement of service users, professionals need to become comfortable with the sharing of knowledge, power and, ultimately, the label of expert.

It is clear that initiatives such as the expert patient programme go some way in challenging both health professionals' and service users' ideas about the role of knowledge and the balance of power between the provider and user of services, but their true potential is as yet unrealised. The aim of user involvement should be to empower service users to question the very existence of services and to reconstruct new ways of working, and this should generate a wealth of possibilities. Tying service user involvement to medical conceptualisations of health, as can be seen in the expert patient programme, will clip the wings before the service user movement has truly learnt to fly. What can be seen to be essential in ensuring that the nature of service user participation can be truly transformative is a shared frame of reference and commitment that ensures that service user involvement is not just acknowledged, but valued and celebrated.

References

Andrews, J., Manthorpe, J. and Watson, R. (2004) 'Involving older people in intermediate care', *Journal of Advanced Nursing*, 46(3): 303–10.

Bailey-McHale, J. (2008) 'Diversity', in E. Mason-Whitehead, A. McIntosh, A. Bryan and T. Mason (eds) *Key Concepts in Nursing,* London: Sage, pp. 109–14.

Bradshaw, P.L. (2008) 'Service user involvement in the NHS in England: genuine user participation or a dogma-driven folly?', *Journal of Nursing Management*, 16(6): 673–81.

Brown, W. and Kandirikirira, N. (2007) *Recovering Mental Health in Scotland: Report on Narrative Investigation of Mental Health Recovery.* Glasgow: Scottish Recovery Network.

Coulter, A. (1999) 'Paternalism or partnership?', *British Medical Journal*, 319: 719–20.

Department of Health (DH) (1999) *Our Healthier Nation – Saving Lives.* London: Department of Health.

Department of Health (DH) (2000) *The NHS Plan: A Plan for Investment, a Plan for Reform.* London: Department of Health.

Department of Health (DH) (2001) *The Expert Patient: A New Approach to Chronic Disease Management for the 21st Century.* London: Department of Health.

Department of Health (DH) (2002a) *Involving Patients and the Public in Health Care.* London: Department of Health.

Department of Health (DH) (2002b) *Shifting the Balance of Power: The Next Steps.* London: Department of Health.

Department of Health (DH) (2004) *The Health Improvement Plan: Putting People at the Heart of Services.* London: Department of Health.

Department of Health (DH) (2005) *Creating a Patient Led NHS.* London: Department of Health.

Department of Health (DH) (2007) *Putting People First – A Shared Vision and Commitment to the Transformation of Adult Social Care.* London: Department of Health.

Department of Health (DH) (2008) *High Quality Care for All: NHS Next Stage Review Final Report.* London: Department of Health.

Department of Health (DH) (2009a) *Implementation of the Right to Choice and Information Set Out in the NHS Constitution.* London: Department of Health.

Department of Health (DH) (2009b) *Supporting People with Long Term Conditions: Commissioning Personalised Care Planning – A Guide for Commissioners.* London: Department of Health.

Edwards, K. (2000) 'Service users and mental health nursing', *Journal of Psychiatric and Mental Health Nursing,* 7: 555–65.

Evans, S., Tritter, J., Barley, V., Daykin, N., McNeill, J., Palmer, N., Rimmer, J., Sanidas, M. and Turton, P. (2003) 'User involvement in UK cancer services: bridging the policy gap', *European Journal of Cancer Care,* 12: 331– 8.

Felton, A. and Stickley, T. (2004) 'Pedagogy, power and service user involvement', *Journal of Psychiatric and Mental Health Nursing,* 11: 89–98.

Forrest, S., Risk, I., Masters, H. and Brown, N. (2000) 'Mental health service user involvement in nurse education: exploring the issues', *Journal of Psychiatric and Mental Health Nursing,* 7: 51–7.

Foucault, M. (1972) *The Archaeology of Knowledge.* London: Routledge.

Foucault, M. (1980) 'Truth and power', in C. Gordon (ed.) *Power/Knowledge: Selected Interviews and Other Writings 1972–1977.* New York: Pantheon, pp. 109–33.

General Social Care Council (2002) *Code of Practice for Social Care Workers and Code of Practice for Employers of Social Care Workers*. London: GSCC.

Health Professions Council (2008) *Standards of Conduct, Performance and Ethics*. London: HPC.

Hickey, G. and Kipping, C. (1998) 'Exploring the concept of user involvement in mental health through a participation continuum', *Journal of Clinical Nursing*, 7: 83–8.

Hui, A. and Stickley, T. (2007) 'Mental health policy and mental health service user perspectives on involvement: a discourse analysis', *Journal of Advanced Nursing*, 59(4): 416–26.

Lester, H., Tait, L., England, E. and Tritter, J. (2006) 'Patient involvement in primary care mental health: a focus group study', *British Journal of General Practice*, 56(527): 415–22.

Lewis, L. (2003) 'Shared decision making in psychiatric consultations: the need to bridge the gap between user and provider perspectives', *Mental Health Nursing*, 23(6): 4–6.

Litva, A., Coast, J., Donovan, J., Eyles, J., Shepherd, M., Tacchi, J., Abelson, J. and Morgan, K. (2002) 'The public is too subjective: public involvement at different levels of healthcare decision making', *Social Science and Medicine*, 54: 1825–37.

Lorig, K., Stewart, A., Ritter, P., Gonzalez, V., Laurent, D. and Lynch, J. (1996) *Outcome Measures for Health Education and Other Health Measures*. Thousand Oaks, CA: Sage.

McCormack, B. (2003) 'A conceptual framework for person-centred practice with older people', *International Journal of Nursing Practice*, 9: 202– 9.

Nash-Wong, K. (2006) 'Building the super consumer', *Pharmaceutical Executive*, 26(6): 104–7.

Newman, J., Glendinning, C. and Hughes, M. (2008) 'Beyond modernisation? Social care and the transformation of welfare governance', *Journal of Social Policy*, 37(4): 531–57.

Nursing and Midwifery Council (2008) *The Code: Standards of Conduct, Performance and Ethics for Nurses and Midwives*. London: NMC.

Oxford English Dictionary (2009) 'Patient.' Available at: www.askoxford. com/concise_oed/patient?view=uk [accessed 28 July 2009]

Peterson, K., Hounsguard, L. and Nielson, C. (2008) 'User participation and involvement in mental health rehabilitation: a literature review', *International Journal of Therapy and Rehabilitation*, 15(7): 306–13.

Poulton, B. (1999) 'User involvement in identifying health needs and shaping and evaluating services: is it being realised?', *Journal of Advanced Nursing*, 30(6): 1289–96.

Rhodes, P. and Nocon, A. (1998) 'User involvement and the white paper: a case of throwing the baby out with the bathwater', *Health Expectations*, 1(2): 73–87.

Robert, G., Hardacre, J., Locock, L., Bate, P. and Glasby, J. (2003) 'Redesigning mental health services: lessons on user involvement from the Mental Health Collaborative', *Health Expectations*, 6: 60–71.

Rush, B. (2004) 'Mental health service user involvement in England: lessons from history', *Journal of Psychiatric and Mental Health Nursing*, 11: 313 –18.

Sang, B. (2004) 'Choice, participation and accountability: assessing the potential impact of legislation promoting patient and public involvement in health in the UK', *Health Expectations*, 7: 187–90.

Sawyer, L. (2005) 'An outcome based approach to domiciliary care', *Journal of Integrated Care*, 13(3): 20–5.

Sawyer, L. (2008) 'The personalisation agenda: threats and opportunities for domiciliary care providers', *Journal of Care Services Management*, 3(1): 41–63.

Squire, S. and Hill, P. (2006) 'The Expert Patients Programme', *Clinical Governance*, 11(1): 17–21.

Stickley, T. (2008) 'Should service user involvement be consigned to history? A critical realist perspective', *Journal of Psychiatric and Mental Health Nursing*, 13: 570–7.

Tang, S.Y.S. and Anderson, J.M. (1999) 'Human agency and the process of healing: lessons learned from women living with chronic illness – rewriting the expert', *Nursing Inquiry*, 6: 83–93.

Warne, T. and McAndrew, S. (2008) 'Value', in E. Mason-Whitehead, A. McIntosh, A. Bryan and T. Mason (eds) *Key Concepts in Nursing*. London: Sage, pp. 315–21.

Weedon, C. (1999) *Feminism, Theory and the Politics of Difference*. Oxford: Blackwell.

Wilson, P.M. (2001) 'A policy analysis of the expert patient in the United Kingdom: self-care as an expression of pastoral power?', *Health and Social Care in the Community*, 9: 134–42.

Wilson, P., Kendal, S. and Brooks, F. (2007) 'The expert patients programme: a paradox of patient empowerment and medical dominance', *Health and Social Care in the Community*, 15: 426–38.

Young, A.F. and Chesson, R.A. (2006) 'Stakeholders' views on measuring outcomes for people with learning disabilities', *Health and Social Care in the Community*, 14(1): 17–25.

7 A Values-Based Era in Professional Caring

Jill McCarthy and Sue Grumley

Values-based care heralds a new era in health and social care provision. However, for this care to be successfully implemented nationally, it needs to be underpinned by values-based education with high-quality research playing a strong, supporting role rather than being the sole driver. With values-based care, targets are person rather than organisation-focused which puts the service user at the centre of care delivery. To achieve this, it is recommended that the paradigm shift from evidence to values, which has already begun, is further developed by leaders in the health and social care sectors. Care is not fixed but fluid, developing and improving as new ideas and innovations are initiated. The introduction of values-based care can realistically be achieved by drawing on previous models of presenting health and social care professionals with new and improved methods of care delivery.

Exploiting the Paradigm Shift from Evidence to Values

The concept of evidence-based practice was introduced to the health care system by Professor Archie Cochrane in the 20th century (Cochrane, 1972). It is defined by Sackett et al. (1996: 71) as the 'conscientious, explicit and judicious use of current best evidence in making decisions about the care of individual patients' and is now accepted as the gold standard for clinical practice.

A change of government and, therefore, policy brought about a review of health services in the late 1990s. The white paper, *The New NHS: Modern and Dependable* (DH, 1997), outlined the objectives of setting minimum national standards of care based on guidelines established using the latest scientific evidence. The paper discussed improving quality through collaboration of health and social services, ending the postcode lottery and paved the way for the introduction of clinical governance in 1999 (DH, 1999) by ensuring efficiency and effective use of available resources. The modernisation of the National Health Service augmented the use of evidence-based practice by encouraging research conducted by all professional groups including allied health professions (Chartered Society of Physiotherapy, 2007a) which facilitated the development of integrated care pathways (Middleton et al., 2001) and challenged the efficacy of some commonly used treatments. The evidence upon which practice is based is graded according to its rigour. The United Kingdom grading system grades evidence from 'A-D', with randomised control trials being the most rigorous and, therefore, graded 'A', and expert opinion being considered the least rigorous and rated 'D' (Royal College of Physicians, 2004). As a result, 'health care decisions are increasingly being made on research based evidence rather than expert opinion or clinical experience alone' (Agency for Healthcare Research and Quality, 2008). Evidence-based medicine developed from evidence-based practice and encourages clinicians to integrate their clinical expertise with the best currently available evidence (Sackett et al., 1996), a developmental step that combines the research with that of prior traditional practice.

The introduction of evidence-based practice and evidence-based medicine may be regarded as partially accomplishing the government's agenda of raising standards and providing a quality service, but each focuses upon the evidence and the clinician, yet fails to significantly focus upon the service user. The question has to be posed: has the pendulum swung too far in one direction? Whilst these developments are geared ultimately to the service user, the needs of the service user appear to have taken a retrograde step. Developments such as integrated care pathways have a tendency to encourage a utilitarian view of health care, with the majority of people being catered for to the detriment of a minority (Beauchamp and Childress, 1994). In the present climate, where human rights are acknowledged and considered sacrosanct, a modern health care service must endeavour to recognise the individuality of the service user and provide an individualistic approach. Choice for the service user was initially referred to in the first NHS review, and pinpointed in further reviews; Lord Darzi's report (DH, 2008a) emphasises the point that people want a greater degree of control and influence over their health and health care.

No one would argue with the aspiration to increase standards and quality, a point accepted by professionals and demanded by service users. Nonetheless, the acquisition of evidence for some treatments can be difficult due to ethical issues or lack of publications. Clinicians may have clinical knowledge gained through experience, but under the evidence grading scheme, expert opinion is deemed the least rigorous category of evidence and, therefore, needs to be considered in conjunction with available published evidence. To illustrate this point, published evidence suggests that occupational therapists are 83.6 per cent accurate in predicting the needs of hospitalised service users on discharge (Frankum et al., 1995) and, therefore, the requirement of a pre-discharge home visit could be challenged. Current literature has failed to produce a single comprehensive list of what a therapist would need to assess a service user for to ensure a safe discharge home, and what determines which service users would benefit most from a home visit (Patterson and Mulley, 1999; Patterson et al., 2001). This is of considerable importance, as home visits are expensive in terms of opportunity costs which are defined as whatever is renounced as a consequence of a decision to use a resource in a particular way. (BSU, 2005; Net MBA, 2007)

Vignette 7.1 illustrates how a combination of both evidence-based practice and expert opinion can result in optimum care delivery. With values-based care, the knowledge and skills of experienced health and social care professionals are combined with quality evidence-based practice to provide care that is fitting to each individual as this vignette illustrates.

Vignette 7.1

I am a physiotherapist and I have real concerns in regard to certain limitations I have noticed with evidence-based practice and care delivery, in particular discharge planning. As I am undertaking a part-time MSc degree, I decided to address this issue as part of my research dissertation. Using qualitative research methods, I organised focus groups with therapists involved in discharge planning in order to explore their knowledge of this area and compare this with available literature; thematic analysis was then used to identify themes and, ultimately, develop an algorithm. This algorithm has been introduced into clinical practice to assist the clinical reasoning of junior therapists when deciding who would benefit from a home visit assessment and forecast the needs of service users when planning a hospital discharge.

This example meets the gold standard of utilising evidence-based practice whilst combining this with clinical expertise to ultimately meet the agenda of furthering research and knowledge and delivering best care to service users.

The introduction of integrated care pathways identified standards of treatment that service users could expect as a minimum (Middleton et al., 2001).

The establishment of minimum standards and the encouragement of multi-disciplinary, multi-agency collaboration and communication can only be viewed positively from the service user's perspective as these all improve services. However, it could be suggested that the prescriptive nature of an integrated care pathway, albeit with accepted variations, diminishes the development of the clinical reasoning abilities of clinicians. Thus, they are potentially relegated to act as expensive assistants whilst treating the service users as a homogenous group who do not have individual values, ideals and opinions. It is, therefore, vital that the views and opinions of both service users and health and social care staff are involved in the planning of care delivery, development of services and strategic planning.

Vignette 7.2 demonstrates the difficulty of working with integrated care pathways in certain circumstances. Care pathways provide excellent care for the majority of service users presenting with the necessary condition, however, although variances are allowed for, there are still set criteria to be met and included in the pathway, which a minority of service users may not present with who may still benefit from this care. Professional judgement which includes intuition, as described in Chapter 5, would have benefited the service user described in the following vignette.

Vignette 7.2

I am a 36-year-old staff nurse working in a local hospice and have been using a Care of the Dying Pathway for several years now. Over time, however, I have noticed that whilst the pathway works very well for the majority of patients that I nurse, ensuring that all aspects of their care are considered, a minority of patients simply do not fit into the pathway for various reasons. Whilst the pathway allows for variance and professional judgement, it is still inadequate for certain patients for a variety of reasons. For example, one patient who was transferred to the hospice from a local hospital and was, in my opinion, clearly in the last days of life, did not present with two of the four conditions necessary to be put on the pathway. After discussion with colleagues, it was decided that the patient could not be in the last stages of life as he was not presenting with the necessary conditions stated. None the less, the patient died within 24 hours of being transferred to the hospice. On reflection, I considered that his care would have been more befitting had he fitted into the pathway criteria, for example, frank and open discussions could have taken place with both the patient and his relatives, which did not occur under the circumstances.

Many councils and Primary Care Trusts have encouraged the development of service user groups to act in the capacity of advocate or sounding board for their group of citizens, for example Knowsley Older People's Voice (2009). These groups sit on local committees in order to represent the older people's views for their particular area. They have been instrumental in challenging strategic plans and modifying local services in response to the needs of their community. Collectively, they play an important role in providing information which can influence developments at a national level, for example attendance at consultation events for the Dementia Strategy.

Since the initial review of the NHS and Social Services in 1997, a further review conducted by Lord Darzi expanded upon the idea of integrating health and social services, recognising that these organisations needed to be more responsive to service users, requirements at both a national and local level. His report *High Quality Care for All – NHS Next Stage Review* (DH, 2008a) builds upon earlier documents, for example *Our Health, Our Care, Our Say* (DH, 2006) and reiterates the importance of increasing quality, whilst establishing the ideas of safe, personalised services, public well-being and prevention services and, primarily, a service with greater choice: 'An NHS that gives patients and the public more information and choice, works in partnership and has quality at its heart' (DH, 2008a: 7).

These recent documents have not dismissed the ideals of evidence-based medicine and practice, but are encouraging the integration of these principles alongside choice for the service user and a more personalised or individualised approach rather than a utilitarian one. These views embrace the concept of a values-based approach to care, initially introduced within mental health services in the United Kingdom, as discussed later in the chapter. The popularity of values-based care is increasing and the concept spreading to physical health services in this country; it has also been introduced into the health care system in the USA. In the American system, information surrounding values-based care refers to quality, but has an overt link to finances and the rising cost of health care (Kahan, 2008), indicating that evidence-based care may be providing unnecessary care on occasions and, therefore, unnecessary expenditure.

Within the British system, values-based care establishes standards for health and social care professionals but clear links to the financial aspects of care are obscured. This would appear to be an oversight considering that the annual cost of funding the National Health Service in 2007 was £90 billon (NHS Choices, 2008).

It has been suggested that within values-based care there are three main areas to consider:

1. Fostering equality and diversity
2. Fostering people's rights and responsibilities
3. Maintaining confidentiality of information
   (Lewisham Council, 2008).

Woodbridge and Fulford (2003) and Petrova et al. (2006) are less specific and advocate that values-based care must address the need to tailor care to the individual, including their beliefs, morals and lives. These views are in alignment with those of Lord Darzi (DH, 2008a) and are facilitating a paradigm shift from evidence-based practice towards values-based care for UK service users.

Today's service user has been encouraged to have greater expectations from the NHS, beginning with the Patients Charter, introduced in 1991. This charter, in conjunction with greater availability of information via the internet, has led to more knowledgeable service users who are not as passive in their acceptance of 'doctor knows best' and will often challenge their local Primary Care Trust, fighting for what they see as their entitlement. For example, stories have hit the headlines of women, diagnosed with breast cancer, who have courted publicity in their fight to secure funding for drugs such as Herceptin, from their local Primary Care Trusts (Dorothy Griffiths Breast Cancer Appeal Fund, 2006).

This signifies a change in the doctor/patient relationship from one that is paternalistic to one that is more equitable and, therefore, a partnership. *Our Health, Our Care, Our Say* (DH, 2006) outlines the requirement to design services to meet the needs of the local population by actively encouraging public engagement and researching service users' experiences and using these as drivers for change in services provided. However, to realise these objectives requires that the service user actively take up this challenge. One of the ways in which service users have become involved is by training to become an 'expert patient'; local government-funded courses run over six weeks educate the service user to self-manage their condition. Research findings of the Expert Patients programme (2008) have demonstrated an improved patient/ doctor relationship, a reduction in Accident and Emergency attendances and general practitioner consultations, and an increase in pharmacy attendances (DH, 2007). These service users are empowered to take control of their conditions and, working in conjunction with their medical and social care team, determine what is in their best interests and what suits their views, lifestyles and ethical beliefs. Recognition of service users' individuality is integral to a values-based approach and a foundation stone of Lord Darzi's review (DH, 2008a). As individuals, we make choices that suit our lives, views and beliefs; as professionals, it is important not to judge other people's standards by our own as they may well differ.

Vignette 7.3 illustrates a situation where a service user's values differ from those of a professional carer and how these were overcome. With values-based care, the values of both the professional carer and the service user are taken into account which can on occasions lead to tensions, however these can be tackled by referring to ethical values, such as patient autonomy, as demonstrated in the following vignette.

Vignette 7.3

I am a district nurse and have been asked to assess a patient who was discharged from hospital following abdominal surgery and requires staples to be removed from the wound area. On arrival at the house, I notice that the standard of cleanliness is poor with stacks of unwashed dishes in the kitchen and the lounge carpet covered in dog hair and dog excrement from a recently purchased puppy that is being house trained. Although I am concerned that the service user's wound does not become infected, I am aware that the service user will have built up a certain immunity to the pathogens within the house and that even the cleanest-looking houses may contain germs that can spread diseases. I caution the service user in regard to cleanliness of the wound area whilst it is still healing and the importance of hand washing before touching or bathing this area. I reflect that it is not my business to comment upon the cleanliness of a service user's house unless they are seriously at risk of harm and that this would simply be judgemental on my part and irrelevant to my care role.

In a democratic society, we have choices, but along with this freedom comes a responsibility for those choices and the consequences which occur as a result of the choices made. For example, diabetic service users who are diet-controlled and choose to consistently imbibe food or drink that is not recommended, have to accept responsibility for their actions and how this impacts upon their health. It is this culture of accepting an individual's right to equitable treatment, whilst acknowledging their diversity, which is becoming the focus for change in health and social care services. The NHS is endeavouring to switch the emphasis from a service that primarily provides treatment, to a system that positively encourages well-being, with an emphasis on the fact that prevention is better than cure. This may present a challenge to some professionals, as it involves a major change to both culture and mindset. As undergraduates in the health and social care professions learn about lifestyle choices and the inevitable consequences of these, so they will realise that the direction taken to date in care has been in regard to dealing with these consequences that are now presenting as health problems. Obesity is reaching epidemic proportions within the UK, not only within the adult population, but also significant rises in childhood obesity have been observed (DCSF, 2008). Research has linked obesity to cardiovascular problems and an increased use of health services. The education of service users around food consumption and exercise has not proved adequate to reduce the levels of obesity within the UK as this also seems to require a shift in culture. Examples of successful cultural changes in regard to diet and lifestyle can be seen through local initiatives. For example, NHS Knowsley has set up a vegetable van that stops within different districts selling affordable fruit and vegetables to Knowsley residents, in an attempt to change the dietary habits and therefore improve the health of the local population (North West Food and Health Taskforce, 2006).

The challenge to health and social care professionals is to alter the approach to care and to seize the values-based initiative by decreasing the emphasis on 'fixing problems' and becoming involved with service users at the very onset of challenges. Using education to prevent escalation of complications rather than the current model of crisis intervention is preferable on many levels. Health and social care professionals are best placed to assist with the development of skills in order that service users may participate in new developments within health and social care services. Some work has already commenced in this area with the introduction of community matrons, whose role involves managing patients with long-term conditions. Their aim is to maintain the service user within their own home environment, to minimise hospital admissions and to facilitate prompt and timely hospital discharges. Many health and social care professionals have knowledge that could promote well-being within local populations, but this requires tapping into. If this challenge is accepted, it could prove to be a pivotal moment for health and social care professionals, opening up more avenues for development, career opportunities and more job opportunities for newly qualified graduates who are currently in plentiful supply in many of the professions (Chartered Society of Physiotherapy, 2007b).

Social Services are moving towards a policy of personalised budgets for service users, giving them more control over the services they receive (DH, 2008b). Currently on discharge from hospital, service users requiring social care receive an assessment of their needs; some of the needs identified may be met by a care package provided by Social Services. Within the current social care system, home care workers have to adhere to an allotted time for each service user within the core working hours of 8.00am to 8.00pm, which can result in some service users becoming dependent rather than encouraging independence. For example, if home carers are only allocated 30–45 minutes for a breakfast call (in which they have to ensure the service user is out of bed, washed, dressed, toileted and fed), those service users who slowly dressed themselves whilst in hospital may not be afforded the time they need. To ensure the completion of the task, the home carer may take on the dressing process and inevitably create a dependency due to the limited time factor.

However, service users who have moved from 'regular' Social Services input to direct payment schemes, have the flexibility to employ their own carers, at a time that suits them and for the period of time they have been assessed for. This process is the precursor to personalised budgets which are currently being piloted around the UK (DH, 2008c). Personalised budgets will ensure that service users have their needs addressed as individuals, therefore reducing the potential of inequalities arising due to disability, race, gender and age, and is truly client-centred and values-based. It is anticipated that personalised care will give the service user access to timely appropriate help and support that is responsive to needs, but is also empowering. This can be achieved by focusing on the prevention of complications for the service user and the promotion of achieving maximum potential (DH, 2008b, 2008c).

Values-based care can be viewed as a tool to improve the quality of care provided by health and social care staff whilst highlighting interventions that do not add value to a service user's life. The effectiveness of an intervention has for the last 30 years been measured in quality-adjusted life years (QALYs) (Sassi, 2006). The QALY assists health care planners and commissioners of services to conduct a cost-effectiveness analysis of an intervention, thus aiding the decision-making process, as resources have a finite limit. Analysis of a situation may identify that some interventions are not cost-effective or could be carried out by working in partnership with others, or by devolving responsibility for the intervention to another agency. This approach has included the independent sector working on NHS waiting-list initiatives, the voluntary sector supporting service users on discharge from hospital (DH, 2004a) and the pooling of budgets and integration of health and social care services (DH, 2005a).

To summarise, the challenge ahead for health and social care staff is to embed the values-based care approach, with its respect for individuals, views, choices and rights, into their working practices. The combination of values-based care and evidence-based practice will ensure a modern, effective approach to health and social care delivery, where the service user shares responsibility for maintaining their own health and well-being, albeit with the help and support of public services. As health and care services start to be designed to suit the needs of local populations, they will differ from region to region across the country, changing to constantly meet the requirements of the communities they serve.

Implementing Values-Based Care

It would appear that a change in the culture of health and social care organisations is required in order to ensure that the challenges of the future are adequately met. People are living longer and it can be reasoned that society has a responsibility to ensure that this results in more years of health and well-being. It is projected that people over 65 years of age with long-term conditions will double over the next ten years and that there will be twice as many people over the age of 85 by the year 2020 (Dunnell, 2007). Therefore, it would seem that a change in how services are delivered is essential as, already, demands for new and improved services are constant. Values-based care may meet this need to some degree as it acknowledges diversity by embracing the values and opinions of the service user when making care decisions and when planning care delivery. Married to this are the values, experience and knowledge of the care professional and thus decisions are made and care delivery provided which is bespoke to each service user.

Ashford et al., (1999: 14) stated that changes in clinical practice were due for a number of reasons:

- variations in practice
- new technologies and advances in professional knowledge
- new evidence from research
- environmental pressures including economic, political and social factors.

It would appear that the drive towards values-based care is emanating from all four of these factors. Service users are no longer passive recipients of care as may once have been the case. Many service users are expert patients and know as much, if not more, about their condition as the professionals involved in treating them (DH, 2007). Today's service users may be more assertive than in the past and often expect and demand the best from health and social care services. They want their voice to be heard and their values to be taken into account when care needs are assessed and care options decided upon. This is recognised in some government benefits which are paid directly to the service user, enabling them to purchase health and care services directly, thus allowing for greater choice and control.

Likewise, many professionals aware of this change of culture in service users, and also aware of the expert patient, no longer feel comfortable taking the lead role in organising or dictating care delivery. There is a plethora of literature including articles in professional journals and government-produced documents (see, for example, DH, 2004c, *NHS Improvement Plan: Putting People at the Heart of Public Services;* DH, 2006, *Our Health, Our Care, Our Say*) which discuss:

- placing the service user at the centre of care
- regarding the service user as a partner in care
- providing the service user with choices in regard to their care.

However, it would seem that this philosophy is somewhat contradicted with the emergence of guidelines, care pathways and protocols for professionals to adhere to, as these arrange for uniform care provision to some degree and detract from individualised programmes of care.

Implementing values-based care will be neither an easy nor speedy task. The title of Sibbald's (2004) article, 'Shockingly complex: the difficult road to introducing new ideas to critical care', demonstrates how difficult changes to even one area of care delivery can be. Ashford et al. (1999) note how change within health care requires adaptation from both the individual and the organisations involved. The fastest and most efficient mode of implementing values-based care would seem to be through the combined approach of a top-down and bottom-up dispersion of knowledge (Panda, 2007). In this case, the top-down direction needs to come through policies emanating from government departments, whilst the bottom-up approach is through the education of professionals who, when released into the workforce, reinforce the importance of values-based care through their practices and networking.

Rycroft-Malone (2008: 1) suggests that contextual factors such as the 'presence, role, and potential influence of leaders' have an important part to play in influencing an individual's care practice. The role of care managers in impacting upon care practice through such activities as support, policy revisions and auditing is commonly acknowledged (see Gifford et al., 2007). However, care managers also need to be directed towards implementing values-based care and it is through government policies that this can be achieved.

The various government departments are influenced on policy making by advisory panels of experts in that particular field. Texts such as this book, articles in professional journals and websites, and presentations at relevant conferences all inform key authorities of the importance of new modes of care delivery. Representatives from respected bodies in the field of health and social care, such as the General Medical Council, the Nursing and

Midwifery Council and the General Social Care Council advise the government in regard to care policy. Word of mouth and the written word influence and inform and, as this information becomes accepted and mainstream through academic and professional debate, it is transferred into documents and policies in order to direct care practices. Values-based care has already taken a foothold in care delivery, especially in mental health services (Petrova et al., 2006) due, in part, to a dissatisfaction with evidence-based care as it lacks true acknowledgement of diversity and difference. Likewise, there has been an interest in values-based practice in primary care settings due to its consideration of individual values. Department of Health policies such as *The Ten Essential Shared Capabilities: A Framework for the Whole of the Mental Health Workforce* (2004b) and *New Ways of Working for Psychiatrists: Enhancing Effective, Person-centred Services through New Ways of Working in Multidisciplinary and Multiagency Contexts* (2005b) are already beginning the drive towards values-based care.

The implementation of values-based care may be viewed as a complex activity which, whilst requiring organisational investment, is reduced to the participation of individual care workers. Ashford et al. (1999) note how resistance to change in health care organisations is pronounced as these are bureaucratic structures which do not easily embrace change. They also note that health care workers are reluctant to change behaviours as they are concerned that they do not harm those in their care and, therefore, prefer tried-and-tested practices. Grimshaw (2007) stated that dissemination and implementation are both human enterprises that can be studied to understand and improve approaches. At the organisational level, effective individual care can be implemented through the various care providers by developing leadership capacity in key individuals at multiple levels within their organisations. In this way, key workers can support colleagues and regulate systems and processes which will encourage the routine use of values-based care throughout their organisations. For example, clinical guidelines supporting values-based care can be produced and it is the responsibility of the organisation to provide these and of the individual worker to adhere to them. A robust system of values-based leadership within organisations can drive the philosophy forward through direct and indirect influences, as care managers are in a strategic position to encourage and enable values-based care.

Vignette 7.4 provides an example of how values-based care can be disseminated amongst colleagues through formal networking channels. Good practice can be adopted through informal methods such as observation, informal discussions and networking and through more formal methods such as education, staff updates and in-house training, as exampled in this vignette.

Vignette 7.4

Julie is a third-year student speech and language therapist who is presently undergoing a practice placement within a hospital setting. Her mentor David, an experienced speech and language therapist who specialises in working with stroke patients, is very impressed with Julie's clinical practice and the way in which she places service users at the centre of care delivery. He has had several service users and staff comment to him about what a caring and professional student Julie is. As he is an advocate of values-based care, which Julie practises, and he realises that she is very current in this mode of care delivery, he feels that she would be an excellent resource for updating staff within the Speech and Language Centre and the Stroke Unit. Therefore, he asks Julie if she would be willing to give an interprofessional presentation about values-based care to some of the qualified and support care staff who work in these specialities. Julie states that this is such a huge topic she feels that two 30-minute slots would be preferable and in this way she can introduce values-based care in one session and follow this up with a second session on applying values-based care in everyday practice. David is pleased with this arrangement and goes ahead with making preparations for the presentations.

Introducing such a dramatic change into care delivery will present challenges. However, there are many successful models of behaviour change which can be utilised for introducing values-based care into the health and social care arenas. For example, Ashford et al. (1999: 20) identify a framework for behaviour change strategies which consists of a practical model involving approaches already familiar to health and social care managers, thus ensuring that this can be adopted with confidence.

To illustrate, first, they consider that a rationale for the proposed change is required and from that standpoint the current situation should be reviewed; they state that this will include:

- individual and social factors
- education and levels of knowledge
- organisational factors
- barriers and facilitators
- resources
- external factors.

They then suggest reviewing current literature which examines change from all perspectives – psychological (social and individual), organisational, educational, innovative and communicational – thus gaining an overall picture of the challenge of implementing the new strategy. From this, they propose developing a strategic and realistic plan in order to successfully implement the change. The plan should identify:

- key groups and individuals
- educational strategies
- psychological and social factors
- marketing and dissemination methods
- clarifying ideas regarding:
  - what the change constitutes
  - the goal of the change
  - criteria for achieving the change.

Finally, they suggest that the change is implemented and that audits and evaluations are undertaken in order to assess progress and modify implementations accordingly.

Familiarity with values-based care will do much to integrate it into mainstream care delivery and this can be achieved through health and social care workers being exposed to information about this innovative approach to care. Grol (1990) noted how change is more easily incorporated by individuals if they are working in close collaboration with peers, which is the situation for a large proportion of health and social care workers. With a current emphasis on continued professional development, health and social care professionals are encouraged to actively update their knowledge and this includes researching pertinent information on various aspects of their roles. Advances in information technology, particularly the World Wide Web, have made access to knowledge revolutionary in that it is freely available to the majority of global citizens. In terms of the dissemination of health and social care information, the internet is an excellent and easily available portal for dispersing information in regard to care issues. There are numerous health and social care websites which promote information in regard to care, for example the Royal College of Nursing and the General Social Care Council, and these can provide a portal for discussions relating to values-based care and, eventually, actively promote this style of care when professional debate on the topic has been fully engaged with.

The Cochrane Effective Practice and Organisation of Care Group (as discussed in Grimshaw, 2007) reviews interventions to improve health care delivery and these reviews fall into four categories:

1. Professional interventions
2. Financial interventions
3. Organisational interventions
4. Regulatory interventions.

This neatly categorises new interventions in care delivery under four umbrella headings. In order that values-based care can be implemented quickly and successfully, it would seem that all four of these interventions will be involved as this is such a massive undertaking affecting all domains of care delivery; some of these have already been touched upon within the chapter. Financial interventions will involve funding for values-based care implementation and financial rewards for staff in regard to this. This may, initially, seem inappropriate as it would appear that rewarding health and care staff for undertaking duties commensurate with their role is immoral. However, it is common for professional development courses for health and social care staff to be paid for by the organisation concerned, in order that professionals are kept updated and skilled. This may be regarded as a legitimate and moral form of financial incentive, whereby staff could be encouraged and supported to attend study days and courses on values-based care. Likewise, staff could be encouraged to attend programmes of study during working hours which, again, may be regarded as a legitimate and acceptable financial incentive. Progression scales based on qualifications, experience and skills are another example of a financial incentive which may be utilised to improve care delivery, again acceptable and commonplace in its usage.

Listening to the service user

Evidence-based practice is developed from scientific research studies and was previously considered the most appropriate rationale on which to base care delivery. However, numerous qualitative research studies have been carried out which are concerned with service users' feelings and opinions about care delivery (Rosenthal and Shannon, 1997) and several of these have demonstrated dissatisfaction with present care delivery patterns including paternalistic styles of care delivery. Demographic changes in the population forecast that there will be further demands on already overstretched health and care resources. Involving service users in care assessment and care choices can ease the burden on human resources to some degree, whilst providing an improved style of care assessment. Listening to the opinions and values of service users and combining these with the values of the professionals concerned can lead to a more caring and appropriate bespoke service. This in turn can lead to less dissatisfaction with health and social care services by allowing the service user to truly take control of their own care.

Vignette 7.5 illustrates how values-based care can work in practice and how, on some occasions, this can minimise resource allocation. Values-based care places emphasis on the service users' values and, therefore, acknowledges that health care is the responsibility of both the service user and the health and social care services. By accepting the service user as a true partner in care (as opposed to tokenistic references), services are delivered which are tailored to the service user's values and in keeping with their personal health care philosophy where possible. The following vignette clearly illustrates such a partnership, which is a compromise working within health and safety parameters.

Vignette 7.5

Jane is 36 years of age and has a diagnosis of multiple sclerosis. Jane's condition has deteriorated and she is referred to the district nursing services by her general practitioner. She is visited by a district nurse who has recently undertaken a module of study on values-based care as part of her professional development. The district nurse, who in the past would have assessed Jane's needs and suggested a care package for her, instead asks Jane for her opinion of her condition and how this can be managed.

Jane tells the nurse that she has recently had a bout of flu and she feels that this has exacerbated her condition. She has had a similar experience in the past and around two months after the flu episode she went into remission and was able to walk again. Jane states that she can manage at the moment with the aid of a neighbour and her mother, both of whom she has discussed this with. Jane explains to the nurse that if she loses her independence by being reliant on state services then she considers that this is the 'beginning of the end' for her. In her mind she would regard this as a downward spiral. Jane says that as long as her life is 'normal', which she equates with not having professional carers involved, then she feels that she can maintain her dignity and control, and keep her outlook bright. She knows that she would become depressed if professional carers were to visit daily and this would further aggravate her condition.

The district nurse respects Jane's strong value of independence. She states that she will telephone Jane in the following week to make sure that everything is working out satisfactorily and she will explain to the general practitioner about Jane's decision to decline health and social care services.

Two months after the visit to Jane, the general practitioner informs the district nurse that Jane has gone into remission again and had walked into the surgery unaided earlier that week to collect her prescription.

Professional Education in Health and Social Care

Changes in care delivery do not happen overnight, nor should they. Thorough discussions and debates as to the benefit of change have to take place in order that new strategies are developed on a sound basis. However, Grimshaw (2007) states that there is consistent evidence that both health care systems and health care professionals fail to deliver the standard of health care that they aspire to, indicating that change is needed. Values-based care has begun to take a foothold in care delivery, and national training for this in the area of mental health is already taking place (DH, 2004b; Woodbridge and Fulford, 2004). This foundation needs to be exploited, by including values-based care as part of the curricula in the training and education of all health and social care professionals. In addition, Return to Practice courses, professional updates and Continuing Professional Development programmes all need to have values-based care on the agenda. In this way, knowledge is dispersed throughout the professions and across organisations.

Education for values-based care will need to encompass several major objectives in order to ensure that its implementation is as successful as possible. Both care staff and service users need to embrace values-based care and this can only be achieved through a full understanding of the advantages this style of care delivery can offer. The following objectives will assist with the overall aim of successfully implementing values-based care:

- developing full awareness and stimulating interest in issues related to values-based care
- enabling each health and social care worker to acquire the knowledge and skills necessary to deliver values-based care
- creating new behavioural patterns as well as shaping individual, group and organisational attitudes to care delivery.

Pursuing the above objectives requires:

- acknowledgment that values-based care is a fundamental component of care delivery for health and social care professionals
- educating service users in regard to elements of values-based care
- securing public access to information about values-based care
- acknowledging that values-based education is a prerequisite for changing the way in which care is presently delivered.

Educational changes should aim towards making positive changes in society. Besides knowledge and experience, education can also foster humanistic values and attitudes. Sources of inspiration for values-based education can be multifaceted, for example case studies which embrace national and cultural traditions, religion and daily routines. Values-based care education should be aimed at creating a knowledgeable, enlightened health and social care workforce that accepts the importance of values, is capable of understanding and acknowledging other people's viewpoints and understands the importance of sharing the decision-making processes with the service user concerned.

Interprofessional education in regard to health and social care can shape relationships between individuals, organisations and service users. For values-based care to be fully accepted and used, it needs to be regarded not only as an indispensable element of the education system for professionals in these areas, but also as a quintessential component of health and social care delivery. Values-based care could be introduced into interprofessional education, taking the form of scenario-based learning, whereby students across disciplines are given a scenario which they work on together in small groups. In this way, the values of the various professions are brought to the forefront whilst acknowledging service users' values represented within the scenario or by inviting service users to become involved. The inclusion of service users and carers in delivering the health and social care curriculum should be incorporated into all health and social care professionals' education where practical and feasible, as this allows for real insights into practical dilemmas and challenges. This should be a paid service recognising the value of these contributions.

Education on values-based care will also need to include educating service users as to this new style of care delivery, as they are the focus of care delivery. This can be informal education taking place through discussions with professionals during the course of their duties, or more formally through patient networks.

Vignette 7.6 provides an example of education in regard to values-based care for service users. As education in regard to values-based care for professionals will take many forms, both informal and formal, so education for service users will likewise be multi-faceted. The following vignette provides an example of professionals exploiting their surroundings to educate service users in regard to values-based care.

Vignette 7.6

The practice manager of a local health centre is tidying up the notice board in the reception area. She asks the practice nurse if she would take a look at the posters and notices that are displayed there and tell her which she feels are current and relevant and which ones she can take down and dispose of.

(Continued)

(Continued)

The practice nurse does this and then states that she would like to inform the public about values-based care delivery as this is an important innovation within the community. She designs a bright poster on the computer which states quite simply what values-based care is and how the values of service users will be taken into account when decisions are made in regard to care delivery. The poster informs service users where they can obtain further information on this subject and it also mentions the role of advocates in speaking on behalf of more vulnerable service users and provides contact details for this. The poster is then placed in a prominent spot in the waiting room where people visiting the health centre will see it.

Conclusion

This book acknowledges the importance of evidence-based practice in assisting with the provision of high-quality care, however it also recognises how we can move beyond this model of practice into a values-based care delivery system. Evidence-based practice may be regarded as having certain shortcomings, not least its reductionist approach to care which places service users into care categories which can override individual needs, values and desires. Likewise, the values, experience and knowledge of health and social care professionals and service users are regarded as less important than research evidence in care delivery. Reductionism has resulted in a return to task orientation and structured frameworks in health and social care, for example single assessment processes, the nursing process and anatomical and physiological systems assessment, with the resulting depersonalisation of service users.

In contrast, values-based care has an holistic emphasis which values the whole person including emotions, intellect, physical being and social integration. Under this remit, health and social care professionals are encouraged to review both their own values and those of the service user they are caring for when making care delivery decisions. The increased public interest in complementary therapies which emphasise close service user involvement during diagnosis and treatment, demonstrates service users' preference for a partnership and voice regarding their own care.

The pressure on academics to constantly publish research findings and the implications for practice, have been discussed within the book. Likewise, the pressure on practitioners to adhere to evidence-based practice has also been critiqued, including the ability to effectively judge research papers. Whether caring is considered an art or a science and the underpinning philosophies of these have been analysed. Caring is a fundamental value in health and social care provision which may be regarded as having been eroded since the introduction of evidence-based practice. Values-based care places the emphasis back on caring and caring skills through the weight it places on the views of service users and their partnership in care.

Professional practice, including professional judgement, intuition and expertise, has not been embraced since the introduction of evidence-based practice and yet these valuable skills, fostered through experience and education, are an important part of care delivery and could be supported and promoted through systems of mentorship and patronage. Values-based care emphasises the need for professional practice gained through knowledge and experience. The importance of recognising the service user's contribution as a partner in care cannot be understated; service users now have a greater choice and control over care services and the emergence of the expert patient has cemented this partnership. Care which acknowledges and embraces diversity is an absolute necessity and leads to the conclusion that there should be a return to individualised values-based care which takes us beyond the frameworks and protocols brought about with the emergence of evidence-based practice.

Values-based care heralds a new era in health and social care provision. It has already begun and has a strong foothold in both mental health and primary care settings. It is imperative that it gains ground in order that personalised care incorporating high-quality evidence-based research, where appropriate, is afforded to all users of health and social care services. This should be an absolute right of service users and the responsibility of all health and social care professionals to ensure this.

References

Agency for Healthcare Research and Quality (2008) *Systems to Rate the Strength of Scientific Evidence*. Available at: www.ahrq.gov/clinic/epcsums/strengthsum.htm [accessed 28 July 2009]

Ashford, J., Eccles, M., Bond, S., Hall, J.A. and Bond, J. (1999) 'Improving health care through professional behaviour change: introducing a framework for identifying behaviour change strategies', *British Journal of Clinical Governance*, 4(1): 14–23.

Beauchamp, T.L. and Childress, J.F. (1994) *Principles of Biomedical Ethics,* 4th edition. Oxford: Oxford University Press.

BSU (2005) [online image]. Available from http://www.bsu.edu/classes/ flowers ppt509c5/51d002.htm [accessed 28 January 2010]

Chartered Society of Physiotherapy (2007a) *Strategy.* Available at: www.csp. org.uk/director/aboutcsp/whatwedo/strategy.cfm [accessed 28 July 2009]

Chartered Society of Physiotherapy (2007b) *Evidence to the Pay Review Body – 2008 Pay Award.* Available at: www. csp.org.uk/uploads/docu-ments/csp%20prb%20evidence%2020083.pdf [accessed 28 July 2009]

Cochrane, A.L. (1972) *Effectiveness and Efficiency: Random Reflections on Health Services.* London: Nuffield Provincial Hospitals Trust. (Reprinted in 1999 for Nuffield Trust by Royal Society of Medicine Press.)

Department for Children, Schools and Families (DCSF) (2008) *Every Child Matters: Obesity.* Available at: www.dcsf.gov.uk/everychildmatters/ healthandwellbeing/commonhealthissues/obesity/obesity/ [accessed 28 July 2009]

Department of Health (DH) (1997) *The New NHS: Modern and Dependable – Executive Summary.* London: Department of Health.

Department of Health (DH) (1999) *Clinical Governance in the New NHS.* London: Department of Health.

Department of Health (DH) (2004a) *Making Partnership Work for Patients, Carers and Service Users: A Strategic Agreement between the Depart-ment of Health, the NHS, and the Voluntary and Community Sector.* Lon-don: Department of Health.

Department of Health (DH) (2004b) *The Ten Essential Shared Capabilities: A Framework for the Whole of the Mental Health Workforce.* National Institute for Mental Health England and the Sainsbury Centre for Mental Health Joint Workforce Support Unit in conjunction with NHSU. London: Department of Health.

Department of Health (DH) (2004c) *The NHS Improvement Plan: Putting People at the Heart of Public Services.* London: Department of Health.

Department of Health (DH) (2005a) *Supporting People with Long Term Conditions: An NHS and Social Care Model to Support Local Innovation and Integration.* London: Department of Health.

Department of Health (DH) (2005b) *New Ways of Working for Psychia-trists: Enhancing Effective, Person-centred Services through New Ways of Working in Multidisciplinary and Multiagency Contexts (Final Report 'but not the End of the Story').* London: Department of Health.

Department of Health (DH) (2006) *Our Health, Our Care, Our Say: Mak-ing it Happen.* London: Department of Health.

Department of Health (DH) (2007) *The Expert Patients Programme*. London: Department of Health.

Department of Health (DH) (2008a) *High Quality Care for All – NHS Next Stage Review: Final Report*. London: Department of Health.

Department of Health (DH) (2008b) *Transforming Social Care*. London: Department of Health.

Department of Health (DH) (2008c) *Personal Health Budgets*. London: Department of Health.

Dorothy Griffiths Breast Cancer Appeal Fund (2006) *News: Women Fighting for Herceptin*. Available at: www.herceptin.dorothygriffiths-bcaf.org.uk/news.html [accessed 28 July 2009]

Dunnell, K. (2007) 'The changing demographic picture of the UK national statistician's annual article on the population', *Office for National Statistics*. Available at: www.statistics.gov.uk/articles/population_trends/changing_demographic_picture.pdf [accessed 28 July 2009]

Expert Patients Programme (2008) *About Expert Patients. Available at:* www.expertpatients.co.uk/public/default.aspx?load=ArticleViewer&ArticleId=500 [accessed 28 July 2009]

Frankum, J.L., Bray, J., Ell, M.S. and Philip, I. (1995) 'Predicting post-discharge outcome', *British Journal of Occupational Therapy*, 59(9): 370–2.

Gifford, W., Davies, B., Edwards, N., Griffin, P. and Lybanon, V. (2007) 'Managerial leadership for nurses' use of research evidence: an integrative review of the literature', *Worldviews on Evidence-Based Nursing*, 4(3): 126–45.

Grimshaw, J. (2007) 'Improving the scientific basis of healthcare research dissemination and implementation', *Ottawa Health Research Institute*. The Hill Group Conferences. Available at: http://conferences.thehill-group.com/conferences/di2007/dayone/01_Grimshaw.pdf [accessed 29 January 2010]

Grol, R.P.T.M. (1990) 'National Standard Setting for quality of care in clinical practice: attitudes of general practitioners and response to a set of standards', *British Journal of General Practice*, 40: 361–4.

Kahan, S. (2008) 'Creating value-based competition in health care', *Essays on Issues. The Federal Reserve Bank of Chicago*. September, No. 254a.

Knowsley Older People's Voice (2009) *Knowsley Older People's Voice*. knowsley_older_people[1].pdf [accessed 1 December 2009]

Lewisham Council (2008) http://ecs.lewisham.gov.uk/intict/vol4/resources/act29/Care%20value%20base.doc [accessed 20 December 2008]

Middleton, S., Barnett, J. and Reeves, D. (2001) 'What is an integrated care pathway?', *Evidence-Based Medicine*, 3(3): 1–8.

Net MBA (2007) *Opportunity Cost*. Available from http://www.netmba.
     com/econ/micro/cost/opportunity [accessed 20 December 2008]
NHS Choices (2008) *About the NHS*. Available at: www.nhs.uk/nhsengland/
     aboutnhs/pages/About.aspx [accessed 1 December 2009]
North West Food and Health Taskforce (2006) 'Fruit & vegetable vans', The
     Newsletter of the North West Food & Health Taskforce, 3: 5.
Panda, B. (2007) 'Top down or bottom up? A study of grassroots NGOs'
     approach', *Journal of Health Management*, 9(2): 257–73.
Patterson, C.J and Mulley, G.P. (1999) 'The effectiveness of predischarge
     home visit assessment visits: a systematic review', *Clinical Rehabilitation*,
     13: 101–4.
Patterson, C.J., Viner, J., Saville, C. and Mulley, G.P. (2001) 'Too many pre-
     discharge home assessment visits for older people? A postal questionnaire
     survey', *Clinical Rehabilitation*, 15: 291–5.
Petrova, M., Dale, J. and Fulford, B. (2006) 'Values-based practice in primary
     care: easing the tensions between individual values, ethical principles and
     best evidence', *British Journal of General Practice*, 56: 703–9.
Rosenthal, G.E. and Shannon, S.E. (1997) 'The use of patient perceptions
     in the evaluation of health-care delivery systems', *Medical Care*, 35(11):
     NS58–NS68.
Royal College of Physicians. (2004) *National Clinical Guidelines for Stroke,*
     2nd edition. Available at: www.rcplondon.ac.uk/pubs/books/stroke/stroke_
     guidelines_2ed.pdf [accessed 1 December 2009]
Rycroft-Malone, J. (2008) 'Editorial: leadership and the use of evidence in
     practice', *World Views on Evidence Based Nursing*, 5(1): 1–2.
Sackett, D.L., Rosenberg, W.M.C., Gray, J.A., Haynes, R.B and Richardson,
     W.S. (1996) 'Evidence based medicine: what it is and what it isn't', *British
     Medical Journal*, 312: 71–2.
Sassi, F. (2006) 'Calculating QALYs, comparing QALY and DALY calcula-
     tions', *Health Policy and Planning*, 21(5): 402–8.
Sibbald, W.J. (2004) 'Shockingly complex: the difficult road to introducing
     new ideas to critical care', *Critical Care*, 8(6): 419–21.
Woodbridge, K. and Fulford, B. (2003) 'Good practice? Values-based practice
     in mental health', *Mental Health Practice*, 72: 30–4.
Woodbridge, K. and Fulford, K.W.M. (2004) *Whose Values? A Workbook for
     Values-based Practice in Mental Health Care*. London: Sainsbury Centre
     for Mental Health.

Index